# Schema Therapy for Complex Trauma

## An Integrative Guide to Healing Childhood Trauma and PTSD

**Deva Maloney Ventura**

ISBN: 978-1-7641438-1-3
Isohan Publishing

This book is intended for educational and informational purposes only and is not intended to replace professional medical advice, diagnosis, or treatment. The information contained herein should not be used as a substitute for the advice of an appropriately qualified and licensed physician, mental health professional, or other healthcare provider.

The techniques, exercises, and information presented in this book are not intended to create a therapeutic relationship between the reader and the author. Readers experiencing symptoms of trauma, depression, anxiety, or other mental health conditions should consult with qualified mental health professionals for proper assessment and treatment.

All names, characters, case studies, and personal stories used throughout this book are created for illustrative purposes only. Any resemblance to actual persons, living or deceased, or actual events is purely coincidental. These composite examples are based on common patterns observed in clinical practice but do not represent any specific individual's experience or treatment.

While the therapeutic techniques and principles described are based on established research and clinical practice, the specific examples and case studies have been created to demonstrate concepts and should not be interpreted as actual case histories.

# Table of Contents

# Preface

The path that led me to write this book began twenty years ago in a small community mental health clinic, where I first encountered Sarah—a thirty-four-year-old woman who had survived childhood sexual abuse, neglect, and emotional torment. Sarah had tried multiple therapies, taken various medications, and worked with skilled clinicians, yet she remained trapped in patterns that seemed to defy every treatment approach we offered.

Traditional cognitive-behavioral therapy helped Sarah identify her distorted thoughts, but the emotional wounds remained raw. Exposure therapy addressed her specific phobias, but new fears emerged like weeds after rain. Medication managed her depression and anxiety symptoms, but the core sense of being fundamentally damaged persisted. Each therapeutic success felt temporary, overshadowed by the return of familiar patterns—self-harm during stress, choosing partners who mirranted her childhood experiences, and an inner voice so harsh it could silence any progress.

During those early years of practice, I encountered dozens of clients like Sarah. They carried what we now recognize as complex trauma—not the aftermath of a single terrible event, but the accumulated weight of repeated childhood experiences that shaped their very understanding of themselves and the world. These clients challenged everything I thought I knew about therapy and healing.

The traditional diagnostic categories felt inadequate. PTSD criteria captured some symptoms but missed the pervasive identity disturbances, emotional dysregulation, and relationship difficulties that defined these clients' daily experiences. Depression and anxiety diagnoses addressed surface symptoms while the underlying architecture of pain remained untouched. Personality disorder labels often felt more like professional frustration than helpful frameworks.

Schema therapy changed everything. When I first learned about Jeffrey Young's integrative approach, something clicked into place—like finding the missing piece of a puzzle I hadn't realized was incomplete. Here was a framework that recognized trauma's deep developmental impact, one that addressed not just symptoms but the fundamental beliefs and coping patterns that childhood experiences create.

## Why This Book Needed to Be Written

The mental health field has made remarkable advances in trauma treatment over the past three decades. We understand trauma's neurobiological impact in ways previous generations could never imagine. Evidence-based treatments like EMDR, trauma-focused CBT, and somatic approaches have helped millions of survivors reclaim their lives.

Yet a significant gap remains. Most trauma treatments focus on specific incidents or symptom clusters, while complex trauma—the result of repeated childhood experiences—requires approaches that address personality-level patterns and core beliefs about self and world. Schema therapy fills this gap, but most resources remain locked in academic language or professional training contexts.

This book bridges that divide. Mental health professionals need practical guidance for integrating schema therapy principles with complex trauma treatment. Trauma survivors and their families need accessible explanations of how childhood experiences create adult patterns—and how those patterns can change. Both audiences deserve hope grounded in solid science and practical application.

The statistics tell part of the story. Studies indicate that 90% of individuals diagnosed with serious mental illness have experienced significant trauma (1). Childhood trauma increases the risk of depression by 400%, anxiety by 300%, and suicide attempts by 1,200% (2). Yet most training programs provide minimal education about trauma's developmental impact, and many therapeutic approaches remain focused on symptom reduction rather than addressing trauma's foundational effects.

**How to Use This Book for Different Audiences**

This book serves three primary audiences, each with distinct needs and learning styles.

**For Mental Health Professionals:** Each chapter includes professional focus sections with clinical applications, treatment protocols, and supervision considerations. Look for detailed case conceptualizations, intervention strategies, and ethical guidelines specific to complex trauma work. The appendices contain assessment tools, training resources, and research summaries to support your professional development.

Pay particular attention to the supervision notes throughout—complex trauma work challenges even experienced clinicians, and regular consultation becomes essential for both client welfare and clinician well-being. The professional sidebars highlight common pitfalls, ethical considerations, and advanced techniques that require specialized training.

**For Trauma Survivors:** Each chapter includes general reader focus sections with accessible explanations, self-reflection exercises, and practical applications. The case studies demonstrate real examples of healing and growth, while safety considerations help you navigate potentially triggering content.

Use the self-assessment tools to increase your understanding of personal patterns, but remember that self-diagnosis never replaces professional evaluation. The resource sections help you locate qualified therapists and support services in your area.

**For Family Members and Supporters:** Understanding complex trauma's impact helps you provide better support while protecting your own well-being. The relationship sections explain how trauma affects attachment and communication patterns, while the practical exercises offer specific ways to support your loved one's healing process.

Remember that healing complex trauma takes time—often years rather than months. Your patience, consistency, and willingness to learn make profound differences in your loved one's recovery process.

### Content Warnings and Safety Considerations

This book discusses childhood abuse, neglect, sexual trauma, domestic violence, and their long-term effects. While I avoid graphic descriptions, the content may trigger difficult emotions or memories. Several safety considerations will help you engage with this material responsibly.

**Grounding techniques** appear throughout the book. When you notice emotional intensity rising, use the 5-4-3-2-1 technique: identify five things you can see, four things you can touch, three things you can hear, two things you can smell, and one thing you can taste. This simple exercise can help you return to the present moment.

**Professional support** becomes essential when working with trauma material. If you're experiencing symptoms like flashbacks, intrusive thoughts, sleep disturbances, or emotional numbing, seek professional help. The resource sections provide guidance for finding qualified trauma specialists.

**Reading pace** matters more than completion speed. Some readers may need breaks between chapters, while others benefit from reading with a therapist or support group. Trust your internal wisdom about pacing and processing.

**Support systems** provide crucial stability during trauma work. Let trusted friends or family members know you're reading about trauma topics, and arrange check-ins or debriefing conversations as needed.

The journey through complex trauma recovery resembles climbing a mountain with multiple false peaks—moments when you think you've reached the summit, only to discover more terrain ahead. Yet each ascent strengthens your capacity, broadens your view, and brings you closer to the authentic self that trauma may have buried but never destroyed.

Schema therapy offers both map and compass for this journey. The framework helps you understand how early experiences created current patterns, while the techniques provide practical tools for creating change. Most importantly, schema therapy recognizes that healing complex trauma isn't about returning to some previous state—it's about creating a new way of being that honors both your wounds and your strength.

This book represents my conviction that trauma survivors deserve more than symptom management—they deserve the opportunity to thrive. The integration of schema therapy with complex trauma treatment offers pathways to healing that honor both the depth of early wounds and the resilience of the human spirit.

# Chapter 1: What is Complex Trauma

Maria sits in my office, describing a life that seems successful from the outside—a thriving career, close friendships, and a loving partner. Yet beneath this surface stability lies a constant undercurrent of emotional chaos that she's battled since childhood. Simple disagreements with her partner trigger overwhelming fear of abandonment. Success at work feels hollow because her internal voice insists she's fooling everyone. Moments of happiness get interrupted by guilt and the expectation that something terrible will inevitably happen.

Maria's experience illustrates complex trauma—not the result of a single terrible event, but the accumulated impact of repeated childhood experiences that shaped her fundamental understanding of herself, others, and the world. Unlike the dramatic imagery often associated with trauma, complex trauma frequently develops in seemingly ordinary families where emotional needs go unmet, boundaries remain unclear, or caregivers struggle with their own unresolved pain.

**Defining Complex Trauma vs Single-Incident PTSD**

Traditional PTSD diagnosis focuses on responses to specific traumatic events—combat exposure, natural disasters, accidents, or violent crimes. These experiences, while devastating, typically occur against a backdrop of previous psychological stability. The person remembers life before trauma and often maintains a core sense of self that trauma temporarily disrupted.

Complex trauma operates differently. It develops when traumatic experiences occur repeatedly during critical developmental periods, typically in childhood. Instead of disrupting an established sense of self, complex trauma shapes identity formation itself. Children experiencing ongoing abuse, neglect, or household dysfunction don't develop trauma symptoms—they develop around trauma, creating personalities organized around survival in dangerous or unpredictable environments.

The clinical research supports this distinction. Studies by van der Kolk and colleagues demonstrate that adults with childhood trauma histories show different brain activation patterns, hormone regulation, and stress responses compared to those with adult-onset trauma (3). These differences reflect developmental adaptations to chronic threat rather than temporary disruptions to normal functioning.

Consider Michael's story. At age forty-two, he sought therapy for work-related stress. During assessment, he revealed a childhood marked by an alcoholic father's unpredictable rages and a mother who alternated between emotional unavailability and overwhelming anxiety. Michael never experienced what most would consider severe abuse, yet he developed a hypervigilant personality, chronic feelings of inadequacy, and relationship patterns characterized by emotional distancing.

Michael's presentation doesn't fit traditional PTSD criteria because no single event caused his difficulties. Instead, thousands of small experiences—walking on eggshells, managing parents' emotions, receiving inconsistent care— created lasting patterns that affect every aspect of his adult life.

## The Developmental Trauma Spectrum

Complex trauma exists on a spectrum, ranging from obvious abuse and neglect to more subtle forms of developmental disruption. This spectrum helps us understand why some individuals develop serious mental health issues despite appearing to have "normal" childhoods, while others show remarkable resilience despite severe adversity.

**Severe End of Spectrum:** Physical or sexual abuse, severe neglect, witnessing domestic violence, having caregivers with active addiction or serious mental illness. These experiences create obvious trauma symptoms and typically receive clinical attention.

**Moderate Spectrum:** Emotional abuse, inconsistent caregiving, parentification (children caring for parents), family secrets, frequent moves or disruptions. These experiences may not be recognized as traumatic but create significant developmental impact.

**Subtle End of Spectrum:** Emotional unavailability, perfectionist expectations, lack of emotional attunement, dismissive responses to child's needs. These experiences often go unrecognized but can create lasting patterns of self-doubt and relationship difficulties.

Understanding this spectrum helps explain why trauma responses vary so widely. Two children experiencing similar abuse may develop completely different coping strategies based on factors like temperament, available support, and other life circumstances. Similarly, children experiencing less obvious trauma may develop significant symptoms if they're particularly sensitive or lack protective factors.

**Neurobiological Impact of Repeated Childhood Trauma**

The developing brain adapts to environmental demands, creating neural pathways optimized for survival in specific circumstances. Children experiencing repeated trauma develop brains wired for threat detection, emotional dysregulation, and survival-focused decision making.

Research by Teicher and colleagues shows that childhood trauma affects brain structure in measurable ways (4). The amygdala—responsible for threat detection—becomes hyperactive, while the prefrontal cortex—responsible for emotional regulation and executive functioning—shows decreased activation. The hippocampus, crucial for memory formation and integration, often shows structural changes that affect how traumatic memories get processed and stored.

These brain changes aren't permanent damage—they represent adaptive responses to dangerous environments. However, they create challenges when individuals try to function in safer adult environments. The brain that helped a child survive an unpredictable home may create difficulties in stable adult relationships.

The hormonal system also adapts to chronic stress. The hypothalamic-pituitary-adrenal (HPA) axis, which regulates stress responses, often becomes dysregulated. Some trauma survivors develop chronic hyperarousal—constantly scanning for threats and reacting intensely to minor stressors. Others develop hypoarousal—emotional numbing and disconnection that provided protection during childhood but creates relationship difficulties in adulthood.

**Case Study: Sarah's Story - Recognizing Complex Trauma Patterns**

Sarah first sought therapy at age twenty-eight for depression and anxiety, but her symptoms didn't respond to standard treatments. Antidepressants provided minimal relief, and cognitive-behavioral therapy helped temporarily before old patterns returned. Previous therapists focused on her symptoms—the panic attacks, depressive episodes, and relationship difficulties—without recognizing the underlying complex trauma patterns.

Sarah grew up in a middle-class family that appeared functional from the outside. Her father worked long hours at a demanding job, while her mother managed the household and cared for Sarah and her younger brother. To neighbors and extended family, they seemed like a normal, successful family.

Behind closed doors, life felt chaotic and unpredictable. Sarah's father struggled with undiagnosed depression and explosive anger. He would arrive home exhausted and irritable, and minor incidents—spilled milk, loud television, normal childhood behavior—could trigger screaming outbursts. Sarah learned to monitor his mood constantly, becoming hypervigilant to subtle signs of his emotional state.

Her mother, overwhelmed by her husband's emotional volatility and her own anxiety, became emotionally unavailable. She went through the motions of caregiving—preparing meals, helping with homework, managing schedules—but rarely engaged emotionally with her children. When Sarah tried to share feelings or concerns, her mother would minimize them or redirect attention to practical matters.

Sarah's brother coped by becoming the family entertainer, using humor and charm to defuse tension. Sarah developed a different strategy—she became the responsible one, managing household tasks and anticipating family needs. This role earned her parents' approval but required suppressing her own emotional needs.

By adolescence, Sarah had developed several trauma-related patterns that would persist into adulthood:

- **Hypervigilance:** Constantly monitoring others' emotional states and trying to prevent conflict

- **Emotional suppression:** Minimizing her own feelings and needs to maintain family stability

- **Perfectionism:** Believing that mistakes would result in rejection or abandonment

- **Caretaking:** Feeling responsible for others' emotions and well-being

- **Identity confusion:** Having little sense of her authentic self beyond her family role

These patterns served protective functions during childhood but created significant difficulties in adult relationships and self-care. Sarah struggled with intimate relationships because she couldn't stop monitoring her partner's moods or suppressing her own needs. Career success felt hollow because she constantly feared being "found out" as inadequate. Friendships remained superficial because Sarah focused on giving support rather than receiving it.

Traditional therapy approaches missed these underlying patterns because they focused on surface symptoms rather than the developmental adaptations that created them. Sarah's depression and anxiety were symptoms of much deeper disruptions to her sense of self and capacity for healthy relationships.

## How Complex Trauma Differs from Other Mental Health Conditions

Complex trauma often gets misdiagnosed because its symptoms overlap with many other mental health conditions. Understanding the differences helps explain why standard treatments sometimes fail and why trauma-informed approaches become necessary.

**Depression:** While trauma survivors often experience depressive symptoms, the underlying dynamics differ significantly. Traditional depression may respond well to cognitive restructuring and behavioral activation. Complex trauma-related depression often stems from deep shame, identity disturbances, and learned helplessness that require specialized approaches.

**Anxiety Disorders:** Trauma-related anxiety typically involves hypervigilance and threat-scanning behaviors that served protective functions during childhood. Standard anxiety treatments focusing on thought challenging may miss the adaptive nature of these responses and the need to address underlying safety concerns.

**Personality Disorders:** Many complex trauma presentations get labeled as personality disorders, particularly borderline personality disorder. While there's significant overlap, the trauma lens emphasizes that "personality" patterns often represent developmental adaptations rather than fixed character traits. This distinction affects treatment approach and prognosis.

**Substance Abuse:** Trauma survivors often use substances to manage overwhelming emotions, intrusive memories, or chronic pain. Treating addiction without addressing underlying trauma frequently results in relapse because the substances served essential self-regulation functions.

**Eating Disorders:** Complex trauma frequently contributes to eating disorders through multiple pathways—using food to self-soothe, control as a response to powerlessness, or body dissociation following abuse. Treatment requires addressing both the eating behaviors and the underlying trauma patterns.

The key difference lies in understanding symptoms as adaptations rather than pathology. This shift in perspective opens possibilities for healing that honor both the survival value of trauma responses and the need for growth beyond survival mode.

### Assessment Tool: Complex Trauma Self-Assessment Checklist

The following questions help identify potential complex trauma patterns. This tool is designed for self-reflection and clinical screening—it doesn't replace professional assessment but can guide conversations with mental health providers.

**Childhood Environment Factors:**

- Did you often feel unsafe or unable to predict what would happen in your family?

- Were your emotional needs consistently dismissed, minimized, or ignored?

- Did you often feel responsible for managing adults' emotions or problems?

- Were there family secrets you had to keep or roles you had to play to maintain stability?

- Did caregivers struggle with addiction, mental illness, or domestic violence?

**Current Emotional Patterns:**

- Do you experience emotions as overwhelming, unpredictable, or dangerous?

- Do you often feel empty, numb, or disconnected from your feelings?

- Are you extremely sensitive to criticism or perceived rejection?

- Do you struggle with chronic shame or feeling fundamentally flawed?

- Are your emotions often confusing or contradictory?

**Relationship Patterns:**

- Do you fear abandonment while simultaneously pushing people away?

- Do you often feel responsible for others' emotions or problems?

- Do you struggle to maintain appropriate boundaries in relationships?

- Do you frequently choose partners who recreate familiar but unhealthy dynamics?

- Do you feel like you're performing a role rather than being authentic in relationships?

**Self-Concept and Identity:**

- Do you have a stable sense of who you are across different situations?

- Do you often feel like you're fooling people about your competence or worth?

- Are you extremely self-critical or have a harsh internal voice?

- Do you struggle to identify your own wants and needs?

- Do you feel fundamentally different from other people?

**Coping and Functioning:**

- Do you use substances, food, work, or other behaviors to manage emotions?

- Do you engage in self-harm or have thoughts of suicide during times of stress?

- Do you experience memory problems or periods of feeling disconnected from yourself?

- Do you have difficulty with sleep, concentration, or decision-making?

- Do you often feel like you're just surviving rather than living?

Positive responses to multiple questions suggest potential complex trauma patterns that warrant professional exploration. Remember that complex trauma exists on a spectrum—you don't need to experience severe abuse to develop trauma-related patterns that affect your life.

Complex trauma recognition represents the first step toward healing. Unlike single-incident trauma, which disrupts an established sense of self, complex trauma shapes identity formation itself. This understanding transforms how we approach treatment—instead of trying to return to a previous state of functioning, we focus on creating new patterns that support authentic self-expression and healthy relationships.

The brain's neuroplasticity means that patterns developed in childhood can change throughout life. The same adaptive capacity that helped you survive difficult circumstances can help you create new ways of being that serve your current life rather than your childhood survival needs.

Schema therapy provides a roadmap for this transformation by identifying specific patterns (schemas), understanding how they developed, and offering practical tools for change. The following chapters will explore this framework in detail, always remembering that your trauma responses represent intelligence and adaptation—strengths that can be redirected toward creating the life you truly want.

**Bridging Forward**

Understanding complex trauma provides the foundation for everything that follows in this book. As we move into exploring schema therapy's framework, remember that recognizing trauma patterns isn't about pathologizing your past or present—it's about understanding how your mind and body adapted to protect you. These adaptations, while they may create challenges now, represent the remarkable resilience of the human spirit.

The next chapter introduces schema therapy as a framework specifically designed to address the deep patterns that complex trauma creates. Unlike approaches that focus primarily on symptoms, schema therapy recognizes that lasting change requires addressing the core beliefs and coping strategies that childhood experiences formed.

**Key Insights from Understanding Complex Trauma**

- Complex trauma develops from repeated childhood experiences rather than single incidents

- The developing brain adapts to environmental demands, creating survival-focused neural pathways

- Trauma responses represent intelligence and adaptation, not pathology or weakness

- Current symptoms often reflect childhood survival strategies that no longer serve adult life

- Healing requires addressing underlying patterns rather than just managing surface symptoms

- Recognition of trauma patterns opens possibilities for creating new ways of being

- The brain's capacity for change means childhood patterns can transform throughout life

# Chapter 2: Introduction to Schema Therapy

The first time I explained schema therapy to David, a thirty-five-year-old engineer who had tried multiple therapeutic approaches, his response was immediate and profound: "You mean there's actually a reason I keep doing these things?" David had spent years in therapy working on individual problems—his tendency to choose critical partners, his workaholism, his difficulty expressing emotions—but no one had helped him see the underlying patterns connecting these seemingly separate issues.

Schema therapy offered David something different: a framework that recognized how childhood experiences create lasting patterns that influence every aspect of adult life. Instead of treating each problem separately, schema therapy revealed the common threads weaving through his difficulties—core beliefs about needing to be perfect to earn love, strategies for avoiding vulnerability, and ways of relating that felt familiar even when they caused pain.

This integrative approach, developed by Jeffrey Young in the 1990s, emerged from his recognition that traditional cognitive-behavioral therapy, while effective for many conditions, sometimes fell short with clients who had deeper, more persistent patterns rooted in childhood experiences. Young realized that lasting change required addressing not just thoughts and behaviors, but the fundamental beliefs about self and world that early experiences create.

## Jeffrey Young's Integrative Model

Young's background in cognitive therapy provided a strong foundation in identifying and changing dysfunctional thought patterns. However, his work with clients who had personality disorders and chronic mental health conditions revealed limitations in purely cognitive approaches. These clients could identify irrational thoughts and develop coping strategies, but somehow always returned to familiar patterns.

The breakthrough came when Young began integrating elements from other therapeutic approaches. From psychodynamic therapy, he borrowed attention to unconscious patterns and early relationships. From Gestalt therapy, he adopted experiential techniques that accessed emotions and body sensations. From attachment theory, he gained understanding of how early relationships shape capacity for connection. From cognitive therapy, he retained focus on identifying and changing dysfunctional patterns.

This integration created something new—a therapy that addressed thoughts, emotions, behaviors, and relationships simultaneously. Rather than viewing these as separate domains requiring different treatments, schema therapy recognized them as interconnected aspects of underlying patterns formed in childhood.

The model's effectiveness lies in its recognition that people develop coherent ways of understanding themselves and the world based on early experiences. These patterns—called schemas—operate largely outside conscious awareness but influence every aspect of adult functioning. When therapy addresses schemas directly, changes tend to be more profound and lasting than interventions targeting surface symptoms alone.

**The Four Main Constructs: Schemas, Coping Styles, Modes, and Core Needs**

Schema therapy organizes human psychological functioning around four main constructs that work together to explain how people develop patterns and how those patterns can change.

**Schemas** represent the deepest level of psychological organization—fundamental beliefs about self, others, and the world that develop from childhood experiences. These beliefs operate automatically and feel absolutely true to the person holding them. A schema of defectiveness, for example, creates the unshakeable conviction that something is fundamentally wrong with you, regardless of evidence to the contrary.

Consider Jennifer's experience. Raised by a mother who struggled with severe depression and a father who worked constantly to avoid the family's emotional pain, Jennifer developed a schema of emotional deprivation—the belief that her emotional needs would never be met by others. This schema influenced every relationship she formed. Even when partners offered genuine care and support, Jennifer's schema filtered their actions through the lens of inevitable disappointment, causing her to either desperately cling or preemptively withdraw.

**Coping Styles** represent the three basic ways people respond to schema activation. Surrender involves giving in to the schema and accepting its predictions as inevitable. Avoidance means trying to prevent schema activation through emotional numbing, substance use, or lifestyle choices that minimize triggers. Overcompensation involves fighting against the schema by behaving in ways that contradict its predictions.

Using Jennifer's emotional deprivation schema as an example, surrender might look like accepting that partners will always disappoint her and settling for relationships that confirm this belief. Avoidance might involve staying single or choosing partners who can't provide emotional intimacy, thus preventing the pain of disappointment. Overcompensation might involve becoming extremely demanding of partners or choosing relationships where she provides all the emotional giving, thus controlling the dynamic.

**Modes** represent moment-to-moment emotional states that combine active schemas with current coping responses. Unlike schemas, which remain relatively stable, modes fluctuate based on situational triggers and internal states. The same person might be in a vulnerable child mode when feeling hurt, a punitive parent mode when self-critical, or a healthy adult mode when responding to challenges with wisdom and self-compassion.

Understanding modes helps explain why people can seem like different people in different situations. Jennifer might function competently as a manager at work (healthy adult mode), become desperately clingy when her partner seems distant (vulnerable child mode), and later criticize herself harshly for being "needy" (punitive parent mode). These aren't separate personalities—they're different combinations of schemas and coping responses activated by different circumstances.

**Core Emotional Needs** represent universal human requirements for psychological well-being. Young identified five basic needs: secure attachment, autonomy and competence, freedom to express valid needs and emotions, spontaneity and play, and realistic limits and self-control. Schemas develop when these needs aren't met in age-appropriate ways during childhood.

The genius of this framework lies in recognizing that problematic patterns always represent attempts to meet legitimate needs. Jennifer's clinging behavior reflects a genuine need for secure attachment, while her tendency to choose unavailable partners represents a familiar attempt to meet this need in ways that feel manageable, even if ultimately unsuccessful.

### How Schema Therapy Addresses Complex Presentations

Complex trauma typically creates multiple schemas that interact in complicated ways, making change feel overwhelming and progress unpredictable. Schema therapy's comprehensive framework provides a roadmap for understanding these interactions and prioritizing treatment interventions.

Traditional therapy approaches often address symptoms sequentially—working on depression first, then anxiety, then relationship issues. This approach can feel fragmented because it doesn't recognize how these problems connect at deeper levels. Schema therapy reveals the underlying architecture that creates multiple symptoms, allowing for more integrated and efficient intervention.

Take Robert's presentation. At forty-one, he sought therapy for what he described as "everything falling apart." His marriage was ending, his business was failing, and he was drinking more than ever. Previous therapists had diagnosed him with depression, anxiety, and alcohol abuse, treating each condition separately with limited success.

Schema assessment revealed a more complex picture. Robert's core schemas included defectiveness (believing he was fundamentally flawed), failure (expecting to fail at important tasks), and emotional inhibition (believing emotions were dangerous and should be suppressed). These schemas developed during a childhood with a father who criticized constantly and a mother who demanded emotional suppression in the name of family respectability.

Robert's current problems all stemmed from these interacting schemas. His business struggles reflected his failure schema's self-sabotaging predictions and his defectiveness schema's underlying belief that success would expose his inadequacy. His marriage difficulties resulted from emotional inhibition preventing authentic intimacy and defectiveness creating hypersensitivity to criticism. His drinking served as both an escape from painful schema activation and a way to temporarily access suppressed emotions.

Schema therapy addressed these patterns simultaneously rather than sequentially. Instead of treating depression, anxiety, and addiction as separate conditions, therapy focused on the underlying schemas that created all three problems. This approach proved more efficient because changes in core patterns automatically affected multiple symptom areas.

**Case Study: Marcus's Journey from CBT to Schema Therapy**

Marcus first entered therapy at age twenty-nine following a panic attack that sent him to the emergency room. Initially diagnosed with panic disorder, he began cognitive-behavioral therapy that taught him to identify catastrophic thoughts and use relaxation techniques to manage anxiety symptoms.

The CBT approach helped Marcus understand his panic attacks and provided useful coping tools. He learned that his thoughts about having a heart attack during panic were unrealistic, and breathing exercises helped him regain control during episodes. For several months, his symptoms improved significantly.

However, Marcus noticed that while his panic attacks decreased, other problems persisted. He continued struggling with chronic self-doubt at work, despite receiving positive performance reviews. His relationships remained superficial because he feared that showing vulnerability would lead to rejection. Most troubling, he found himself constantly anticipating the return of panic symptoms, creating a different kind of anxiety that CBT techniques couldn't address.

When Marcus's panic attacks returned during a stressful work period, his CBT therapist increased session frequency and suggested medication. While these interventions provided some relief, Marcus felt frustrated by the cyclical nature of his symptoms. He described feeling like he was "managing" his problems rather than truly resolving them.

A colleague recommended schema therapy, and Marcus decided to try a different approach. The initial assessment revealed patterns that CBT had never addressed. Marcus's schemas included vulnerability to harm (believing danger lurked everywhere), defectiveness (feeling fundamentally flawed), and approval-seeking (needing constant validation from others).

These schemas developed during a childhood with an anxious mother who communicated constant worry about potential dangers and a father who provided love and attention only when Marcus achieved academically or behaviorally. Marcus learned to scan constantly for threats while suppressing any signs of struggle that might disappoint his parents.

Schema therapy helped Marcus understand that his panic attacks represented just one manifestation of deeper patterns. His vulnerability schema created chronic hypervigilance that eventually triggered panic responses. His defectiveness schema made him interpret panic symptoms as evidence of personal weakness. His approval-seeking schema prevented him from seeking support when struggling, increasing isolation and symptom intensity.

Treatment focused on these underlying patterns rather than just panic symptoms. Marcus learned to recognize schema activation in various life situations, not just anxiety-provoking ones. He practiced expressing vulnerability in safe relationships, challenging his belief that showing struggles would result in rejection. Most importantly, he developed a more compassionate relationship with his symptoms, understanding them as protective responses rather than signs of personal failure.

After eighteen months of schema therapy, Marcus's changes extended far beyond panic symptom management. His work relationships improved as he stopped constantly seeking approval and began expressing his authentic opinions. His romantic relationship deepened as he shared struggles and fears rather than maintaining a facade of constant competence. While he occasionally experienced anxiety, it no longer felt overwhelming because he understood its purpose and had tools for responding compassionately.

**Why Traditional Therapy Sometimes Isn't Enough**

Traditional therapeutic approaches often focus on symptom reduction rather than pattern transformation. This approach works well for many conditions, particularly those with clear triggers and specific behavioral components. However, complex trauma creates patterns that operate at multiple levels simultaneously, requiring more comprehensive intervention.

**Cognitive Therapy Limitations:** While cognitive therapy effectively challenges distorted thoughts, trauma-related beliefs often feel absolutely true at emotional and body levels. A person might intellectually understand that not everyone will abandon them while still experiencing overwhelming fear during relationship conflicts. Schema therapy addresses these beliefs at emotional and experiential levels, not just cognitive ones.

**Behavioral Therapy Limitations:** Behavioral interventions can change specific actions but may miss the underlying motivations that drive repeated patterns. A person might learn to stop self-harming during crisis but continue struggling with the emotional dysregulation and shame that originally motivated the behavior. Schema therapy addresses both the behavior and its underlying functions.

**Medication Limitations:** Psychiatric medications can effectively manage symptoms like depression, anxiety, and mood instability. However, they don't address the beliefs, relationship patterns, and coping strategies that complex trauma creates. Many clients benefit from medication as part of comprehensive treatment, but medication alone rarely creates lasting change in trauma-related patterns.

**Short-term Therapy Limitations:** Insurance pressures and clinical training often emphasize brief interventions that focus on immediate symptom relief. While this approach serves many clients well, complex trauma patterns developed over years or decades typically require longer-term intervention. Schema therapy recognizes that deep pattern change takes time and provides framework for sustained therapeutic work.

The integration of multiple therapeutic approaches in schema therapy addresses these limitations by recognizing that lasting change requires intervention at cognitive, emotional, behavioral, and relational levels simultaneously. Rather than viewing different symptoms as separate problems requiring different treatments, schema therapy reveals the underlying patterns that create multiple difficulties and addresses them comprehensively.

**Self-Reflection Exercise: Identifying Your Personal Patterns**

The following exercise helps you begin recognizing potential schema patterns in your own life. Approach this exploration with curiosity rather than judgment—schemas developed as adaptive responses to childhood circumstances and continue because they once served important functions.

**Pattern Recognition Questions:**

*Relationship Patterns:*

- What types of people do you repeatedly attract or feel attracted to?

- What conflicts or disappointments show up repeatedly in your relationships?

- How do you typically respond when relationships become challenging?

- What fears or concerns do you have about being truly known by others?

*Work and Achievement Patterns:*

- How do you typically respond to success and failure?

- What drives you to work hard or achieve goals?

- How do you handle criticism or feedback from supervisors or colleagues?

- What beliefs do you hold about your competence and abilities?

*Emotional Patterns:*

- Which emotions feel most comfortable and uncomfortable for you?

- How do you typically handle strong emotions when they arise?

- What strategies do you use to cope with stress or overwhelm?

- How would you describe your internal voice when you make mistakes?

*Family Background Connections:*

- What messages did you receive about emotions, achievement, and relationships in your family?

- How did family members handle conflict, stress, and emotional expression?

- What roles did you play in your family system (caretaker, performer, problem, etc.)?

- What felt unsafe or unpredictable in your childhood environment?

**Pattern Integration:** After reflecting on these questions, look for themes that connect across different life areas. Schemas typically create consistent patterns that show up in relationships, work, and self-care. For example, a pattern of taking care of others' needs while ignoring your own might appear in romantic relationships, friendships, work dynamics, and family interactions.

Notice how current patterns might have served protective functions during childhood. The hypervigilance that creates anxiety in safe adult situations may have been essential for navigating an unpredictable family environment. The perfectionism that causes stress at work might have been the only way to receive attention or avoid criticism as a child.

Remember that recognizing patterns represents the beginning of change, not an endpoint. Schema therapy provides tools for transforming these patterns while honoring their original protective functions. The goal isn't to eliminate schemas entirely but to reduce their intensity and develop more flexible responses that serve your current life circumstances.

**Understanding Your Adaptive Intelligence**

Schema therapy's foundation rests on recognizing that what we often call "pathology" represents adaptation—intelligent responses to environmental demands that may no longer serve current circumstances. Your brain developed patterns that helped you survive and function in your childhood environment. These patterns represent strengths, even when they create difficulties in adult life.

This perspective transforms the therapeutic process from one of fixing something broken to one of understanding and redirecting existing strengths. Your capacity to develop survival strategies demonstrates the same intelligence that can create new patterns supporting the life you want now.

The framework of schemas, coping styles, modes, and core needs provides a map for this transformation. Rather than viewing your struggles as evidence of personal failure, schema therapy reveals them as logical responses to life circumstances. This understanding opens possibilities for change that honor both your survival intelligence and your growth potential.

As we move forward in this book, we'll explore how trauma specifically creates schema patterns and how those patterns can be transformed through targeted intervention. The foundation we've established here—understanding schemas as adaptive intelligence rather than pathology—will guide every step of the healing process.

**Key Insights from Schema Therapy Foundations**

- Schemas represent intelligent adaptations to childhood circumstances, not personal defects

- The four constructs (schemas, coping styles, modes, core needs) explain how patterns develop and change

- Integration of multiple therapeutic approaches addresses change at cognitive, emotional, and behavioral levels

- Current problems often represent attempts to meet legitimate needs in familiar but ineffective ways

- Pattern recognition provides the foundation for transformation while honoring adaptive intelligence

- Lasting change requires addressing underlying patterns rather than just managing surface symptoms

- Understanding your schemas as survival strategies opens possibilities for creating new patterns that serve your current life

# Chapter 3: The Schema-Trauma Connection

When Lisa first described her childhood, she spoke matter-of-factly about experiences that would horrify most listeners. Her father's drinking binges that lasted for days. Her mother's emotional breakdowns that left Lisa caring for younger siblings at age eight. The unpredictable explosions of rage followed by periods of eerie calm. The constant feeling that something terrible might happen at any moment.

What struck me most wasn't the severity of Lisa's experiences, but her casual tone in describing them. "It wasn't that bad," she insisted. "Lots of kids have it worse." This minimization represented more than simple denial—it reflected how trauma shapes the very framework we use to understand our experiences. Lisa's schemas had organized around the need to survive her childhood environment, creating beliefs and coping strategies that made sense in that context but caused significant problems in her adult life.

The connection between trauma and schema formation represents one of schema therapy's most powerful insights. Unlike other therapeutic approaches that treat trauma and personality patterns as separate issues, schema therapy recognizes that early traumatic experiences literally shape personality development. The beliefs, coping strategies, and relationship patterns that define who we are often develop as direct responses to childhood trauma.

### How Trauma Creates Early Maladaptive Schemas

Schemas form when core emotional needs go unmet during critical developmental periods. While some schemas develop from obvious trauma like abuse or neglect, others emerge from more subtle experiences—emotional unavailability, inconsistent caregiving, or family environments that discourage authentic emotional expression.

The process begins with a child's attempt to make sense of experiences that feel overwhelming or threatening. When a parent responds to emotional needs with irritation or dismissal, the child doesn't conclude that the parent is struggling or unavailable. Instead, the child's developing mind creates explanations that preserve the attachment relationship: "I must be too demanding," "My feelings are wrong," or "I need to be perfect to deserve love."

These conclusions feel logical within the child's limited understanding of relationships and causation. Children naturally assume responsibility for their experiences because accepting that caregivers are flawed or unavailable threatens their sense of safety and security. It feels safer to believe you're defective than to accept that the people you depend on for survival can't meet your needs.

Once formed, schemas operate like invisible filters that shape how new experiences get interpreted. A child who develops a defectiveness schema will interpret neutral feedback as criticism, kind gestures as pity, and success as temporary luck. These interpretations reinforce the original schema, creating self-perpetuating cycles that persist long after the original trauma ends.

Consider Jason's development of an abandonment schema. His mother struggled with severe depression following his father's death when Jason was six. While she never intended harm, her emotional unavailability during this critical period left Jason feeling desperately alone and terrified of losing the people he loved. Every time his mother withdrew into depressive episodes, Jason's young mind reinforced the belief that people he loved would inevitably leave him.

This abandonment schema shaped Jason's entire relational development. In school, he became the class clown, desperately trying to maintain others' attention and approval. In friendships, he gave constantly while asking for little, afraid that expressing needs would drive people away. In romantic relationships, he alternated between clinging desperately and pushing partners away preemptively to avoid the pain of inevitable abandonment.

**The Five Schema Domains and Trauma Types**

Young organized the eighteen early maladaptive schemas into five domains that correspond to different types of childhood experiences and unmet needs. Understanding these domains helps explain how specific trauma types create predictable schema patterns.

**Disconnection and Rejection Domain** develops when children experience environments that feel unsafe, unpredictable, or emotionally cold. These schemas reflect the belief that emotional needs won't be met by others and that relationships are fundamentally dangerous or disappointing.

The abandonment schema emerges when children experience actual or threatened loss of important caregivers. This might result from death, divorce, frequent moves, or emotional unavailability. Children conclude that people they love will inevitably leave, creating hypervigilance about signs of rejection and desperate attempts to prevent abandonment.

Mistrust and abuse schemas develop when children experience betrayal, manipulation, or harm from caregivers or other trusted figures. These schemas create the expectation that others will hurt, humiliate, or take advantage of you. Even in safe adult relationships, these schemas generate constant scanning for signs of betrayal or exploitation.

Emotional deprivation schemas form when children's emotional needs consistently go unmet. This might happen with caregivers who are physically present but emotionally unavailable, or in families where emotional expression is discouraged. Children learn that their emotional needs are unimportant or burdensome to others.

**Impaired Autonomy and Performance Domain** develops when children's independence and competence are either discouraged or demanded prematurely. These schemas reflect beliefs about personal capability and the safety of independent action.

Dependence schemas emerge when children are overprotected or when their attempts at independence are discouraged or criticized. The child learns to doubt their ability to handle normal life challenges without significant help from others. While this might seem protective, it actually creates anxiety and learned helplessness.

Vulnerability to harm schemas develop when children are taught to fear normal life experiences or when they experience traumatic events that create lasting fearfulness. These schemas generate constant anxiety about potential catastrophes and often lead to avoidance of normal life activities.

**Other-Directedness Domain** develops in families where children learn that their own needs, emotions, and preferences are less important than maintaining others' approval or emotional stability. These schemas reflect the belief that love and acceptance depend on suppressing authentic self-expression.

Subjugation schemas form when children learn that expressing their needs or preferences leads to conflict, rejection, or retaliation. To maintain relationships, these children suppress their authentic selves and focus exclusively on pleasing others. This pattern often persists into adulthood, creating relationships characterized by resentment and emotional exhaustion.

Self-sacrifice schemas develop when children become responsible for managing adults' emotional needs or family stability. These children learn that their worth depends on helping others, often at the expense of their own well-being. While self-sacrifice can look admirable, it often reflects trauma-based beliefs about worthiness and safety.

**Impaired Limits Domain** develops when children don't learn appropriate boundaries, self-control, or respect for others' rights. This might happen through overindulgence, lack of consequences, or modeling of entitled or impulsive behavior.

**Overvigilance and Inhibition Domain** develops in families that emphasize control, perfection, and emotional suppression. Children learn that spontaneous expression is dangerous and that they must maintain constant vigilance to avoid making mistakes or losing control.

**Attachment Theory Meets Schema Therapy**

Attachment theory provides crucial understanding of how early relationships shape capacity for connection throughout life. Schema therapy builds on these insights by explaining the specific beliefs and coping patterns that different attachment experiences create.

Secure attachment develops when caregivers respond to children's needs consistently and sensitively. Children with secure attachment learn that relationships can be safe, that their needs matter, and that they're worthy of love and care. These early experiences create schemas that support healthy adult relationships—basic trust, emotional stability, and confidence in their ability to handle life challenges.

Anxious attachment develops when caregiving is inconsistent or when caregivers are struggling with their own emotional difficulties. Children learn that relationships are important but unpredictable, leading to schemas characterized by fear of abandonment, emotional deprivation, and desperate attempts to maintain connection. Adults with anxious attachment often struggle with jealousy, clinging behavior, and emotional dysregulation in relationships.

Avoidant attachment emerges when caregivers consistently reject or minimize children's emotional needs. To maintain some connection, children learn to suppress their needs and emotions, developing schemas of emotional inhibition and self-reliance. Adults with avoidant attachment often struggle with intimacy and emotional expression, maintaining distance to avoid rejection.

Disorganized attachment develops in environments characterized by trauma, abuse, or severely inconsistent caregiving. Children develop contradictory needs for connection and safety, leading to complex schema patterns that might include abandonment fears alongside mistrust, or desperate clinging alternating with emotional withdrawal.

Schema therapy's contribution lies in recognizing that attachment patterns continue influencing adult relationships through specific cognitive, emotional, and behavioral patterns. Rather than viewing attachment styles as fixed categories, schema therapy provides tools for identifying and changing the underlying beliefs and coping strategies that create attachment difficulties.

**Case Study: The Williams Family - Intergenerational Trauma Patterns**

The Williams family story illustrates how trauma patterns pass from generation to generation, creating cycles that feel impossible to break without conscious intervention. Understanding these patterns helps explain why trauma effects persist even when people are motivated to change and why healing often requires addressing family-of-origin experiences.

**Grandmother Margaret's Generation** Margaret Williams grew up during the Great Depression in a family struggling with poverty and her father's alcoholism. As the eldest daughter, she became responsible for caring for younger siblings while her mother worked multiple jobs. Margaret developed schemas of self-sacrifice and emotional inhibition—she learned that her needs didn't matter and that showing emotions was a luxury the family couldn't afford.

Margaret survived by becoming hyperresponsible and emotionally controlled. These adaptations helped her manage an overwhelming childhood, but they also shaped her approach to parenting. She raised her children with the same emotional suppression and responsibility demands that had helped her survive, genuinely believing she was preparing them for a harsh world.

**Father David's Generation** David Williams grew up with a mother who demanded emotional control and premature responsibility. Margaret's trauma-based parenting created an environment where emotions felt dangerous and children's needs seemed burdensome. David developed schemas of emotional deprivation (his emotional needs consistently went unmet) and emotional inhibition (expressing emotions led to criticism or dismissal).

David coped with these schemas through avoidance and overcompensation. He threw himself into academic and career achievement, believing that success would finally earn him the emotional connection he craved. However, his emotional inhibition schema prevented him from expressing vulnerability even when he achieved success, leaving him feeling perpetually empty and disconnected.

When David became a parent, his unresolved schemas created similar patterns for his children. Despite loving them deeply, his emotional inhibition made him emotionally unavailable. His own unmet needs for connection made his children's emotional demands feel overwhelming, leading him to respond with the same dismissiveness he had experienced.

40

**Current Generation: Lisa and Michael** Lisa and Michael Williams grew up with a father who worked constantly and struggled to express emotions, and a mother who was overwhelmed by single-handedly managing the household's emotional needs. While their family appeared successful from the outside, the children experienced emotional neglect that created lasting schema patterns.

Lisa developed schemas of emotional deprivation and self-sacrifice. She learned that her emotional needs were burdensome and that her worth depended on caring for others. As an adult, she found herself in relationships where she gave constantly while receiving little emotional support, recreating the familiar pattern of emotional starvation.

Michael developed different schemas from similar experiences. His coping strategy involved overcompensation—he became extremely successful professionally while struggling with intimate relationships. His achievement temporarily filled the emotional void, but he remained vulnerable to depression and anxiety when work wasn't going well.

**Breaking the Cycle** The Williams family pattern might have continued indefinitely if Lisa hadn't entered therapy following a relationship crisis. Schema therapy helped her understand how her family's trauma history had shaped her beliefs about relationships and self-worth. More importantly, it provided tools for creating new patterns that could break the intergenerational cycle.

Lisa's healing process involved several stages. First, she needed to recognize her schemas and understand their origins without blaming her parents or herself. This required developing compassion for her family's struggles while

41

acknowledging the impact on her development. Next, she practiced expressing emotional needs in safe relationships, challenging her belief that her emotions were burdensome. Finally, she learned to choose partners who could actually meet her emotional needs rather than those who felt familiar but emotionally unavailable.

The changes Lisa made affected not only her own life but also her relationships with family members and her approach to future parenting. By healing her own trauma patterns, she created the possibility of raising children who wouldn't inherit the family's emotional suppression and self-sacrifice patterns.

### Breaking the Cycle of Trauma Transmission

Intergenerational trauma transmission happens automatically when unresolved trauma patterns influence parenting behavior. Parents naturally teach what they learned in childhood, even when they're consciously trying to do better. Breaking these cycles requires conscious intervention that addresses both current patterns and their historical origins.

**Understanding Triggers and Reactions** Trauma-related schemas often get activated during parenting moments that mirror the parent's childhood experiences. A parent with abandonment schemas might panic when their child expresses independence, unconsciously trying to prevent the abandonment they fear. A parent with emotional inhibition schemas might feel overwhelmed by their child's emotional intensity, responding with the same dismissiveness they experienced.

These reactions happen automatically because schemas operate below conscious awareness. The parent isn't choosing to recreate trauma patterns—their nervous system is responding to perceived threats based on childhood learning. Breaking the cycle requires developing awareness of these automatic responses and creating new choices in triggering moments.

**Developing Emotional Regulation Skills** Parents can't teach emotional skills they haven't developed themselves. A parent who learned to suppress emotions during childhood will struggle to help their child process difficult feelings. A parent who never learned to set boundaries will have difficulty teaching their child about limits and self-respect.

Schema therapy emphasizes developing the emotional regulation and relationship skills that trauma may have disrupted. This might involve learning to identify and express emotions, developing self-compassion, or practicing boundary-setting. These skills benefit the parent's own healing while providing a foundation for healthier parenting.

**Creating Repair and Connection** Perfect parenting isn't necessary for healthy child development—responsive repair when problems occur is more important than avoiding all mistakes. Parents who experienced trauma often fear that any mistakes will damage their children irreparably. This perfectionist pressure actually interferes with the authentic connection that children need.

Learning to repair mistakes authentically teaches children that relationships can withstand conflict and that they're worthy of effort and attention when problems arise. A parent who can say "I was overwhelmed and responded harshly, but that wasn't about you" provides a completely different model than the parent who either ignores problems or blames the child for causing them.

### Assessment Tool: Trauma-Informed Schema Assessment

This assessment tool helps identify potential schema patterns that may have developed from childhood trauma. Use it as a starting point for understanding your patterns rather than a diagnostic tool—professional assessment provides more accurate evaluation of complex trauma patterns.

### Disconnection and Rejection Domain Assessment:

*Abandonment Schema Indicators:*

- Do you fear that people you love will leave or die?

- Do you become extremely upset when people are late or cancel plans?

- Do you tend to cling to relationships or push people away when you feel threatened?

- Do you feel desperate when relationships end, even unhealthy ones?

*Mistrust/Abuse Schema Indicators:*

- Do you expect people to hurt, humiliate, or take advantage of you?

- Do you find it difficult to trust others, even when they've proven trustworthy?

- Are you suspicious of others' motives, especially when they're being kind?

- Do you feel like you need to protect yourself from being exploited?

*Emotional Deprivation Schema Indicators:*

- Do you feel like your emotional needs will never be met by others?

- Do you often feel lonely, even in relationships?

- Do you expect others to be emotionally unavailable or uninterested in your feelings?

- Do you rarely share your emotional needs because you assume others won't care?

**Impaired Autonomy Domain Assessment:**

*Dependence Schema Indicators:*

- Do you feel unable to handle everyday problems without help from others?

- Do you worry about your ability to make good decisions?

- Do you rely heavily on others for practical and emotional support?

- Do you avoid challenging situations because you doubt your competence?

*Vulnerability Schema Indicators:*

- Do you worry excessively about potential catastrophes or dangers?

- Do you avoid activities because you fear something bad will happen?

- Do you feel like you're unable to protect yourself from harm?

- Do you experience frequent anxiety about health, safety, or security?

**Other-Directedness Domain Assessment:**

*Subjugation Schema Indicators:*

- Do you suppress your own needs and preferences to avoid conflict?

- Do you feel controlled by others and unable to express your authentic self?

- Do you fear that expressing your needs will lead to retaliation or abandonment?

- Do you often feel angry or resentful but unable to express these feelings?

*Self-Sacrifice Schema Indicators:*

- Do you focus excessively on meeting others' needs at the expense of your own?

- Do you feel guilty when you do things for yourself?

- Do you often feel responsible for others' emotions and well-being?

- Do you have difficulty saying no to requests, even when you're overwhelmed?

**Overvigilance Domain Assessment:**

*Emotional Inhibition Schema Indicators:*

- Do you have difficulty expressing emotions, especially vulnerable ones?

- Do you feel uncomfortable when others express strong emotions?

- Do you believe that showing emotions is a sign of weakness or immaturity?

- Do you often feel disconnected from your emotional experiences?

*Unrelenting Standards Schema Indicators:*

- Do you feel like your efforts are never good enough?

- Do you drive yourself relentlessly to meet extremely high standards?

- Do you focus more on mistakes and flaws than successes and strengths?

- Do you believe that anything less than perfection is failure?

**Trauma History Connections:** After completing the schema assessment, reflect on connections between current patterns and childhood experiences:

- Which schemas feel most accurate for your experience?

- Can you identify childhood experiences that might have contributed to these patterns?

- How do these schemas currently affect your relationships, work, and self-care?

- What coping strategies do you use when these schemas get activated?

Remember that schemas exist on a continuum—you might have mild versions of several schemas rather than severe versions of just one or two. The goal isn't to eliminate schemas entirely but to reduce their intensity and develop more flexible responses when they get triggered.

**The Architecture of Survival**

Understanding the connection between trauma and schema formation reveals the remarkable intelligence of the human adaptation system. Your schemas didn't develop randomly or represent character flaws—they emerged as logical responses to specific environmental demands. The child who developed emotional inhibition in a family where emotions were dangerous demonstrated the same intelligence that can now learn new emotional skills in safer environments.

This perspective transforms healing from a process of fixing something broken to one of understanding and redirecting existing strengths. Your capacity to develop survival strategies reflects the same neuroplasticity that enables creating new patterns supporting the life you want now.

The framework we've established—understanding how trauma creates schemas through disrupted attachment and unmet core needs—provides the foundation for everything that follows in this book. As we explore specific schemas and their treatment, remember that each pattern represents an adaptation that once served important functions. Healing honors both the survival value of these adaptations and your current need for patterns that support thriving rather than just surviving.

Schema therapy's integration of trauma understanding with practical change techniques offers hope for breaking cycles that may have persisted for generations. Your willingness to understand these patterns and work toward change creates possibilities not just for your own healing, but for preventing trauma transmission to future generations.

**Key Insights from the Schema-Trauma Connection**

- Schemas develop as intelligent adaptations to childhood environments, not as character defects

- Trauma creates predictable schema patterns organized around five domains of unmet needs

- Attachment experiences shape capacity for adult relationships through specific cognitive and emotional patterns

- Intergenerational trauma transmission occurs when unresolved patterns influence parenting behavior

- Breaking trauma cycles requires conscious intervention addressing both current patterns and historical origins

- Recognition of schemas as survival adaptations opens possibilities for transformation

- Understanding your patterns provides the foundation for creating new responses that serve your current life rather than childhood survival needs

# Chapter 4: Disconnection and Rejection Schemas

The emergency room nurse looked at Rebecca with skepticism when she arrived for the third time that month, clutching her chest and gasping for breath. "The tests are normal," the doctor explained patiently, "Your heart is fine." But Rebecca's terror felt real—the crushing sensation in her chest, the certainty that something catastrophic was about to happen. She couldn't explain that this wasn't just anxiety about her health. This was the familiar feeling of abandonment that had lived in her body since childhood, now triggered by her boyfriend's casual mention of spending the weekend with friends.

Rebecca's panic attacks represented just one manifestation of deep schemas formed in the first domain of early maladaptive patterns—disconnection and rejection. These schemas develop when children experience environments that feel unsafe, unpredictable, or emotionally barren. The child's fundamental need for secure attachment goes unmet, creating lasting beliefs that relationships are dangerous and that emotional needs will inevitably lead to disappointment or pain.

Understanding these five schemas—abandonment, mistrust/abuse, emotional deprivation, defectiveness, and social isolation—provides a roadmap for recognizing how early experiences of rejection and disconnection shape adult relationship patterns. More importantly, it offers hope for healing wounds that may have felt permanent for decades.

## How Neglect and Abuse Create These Schemas

Children enter the world with an innate expectation that caregivers will provide safety, connection, and emotional responsiveness. This biological programming ensures survival and healthy development. But when this expectation repeatedly goes unmet—through neglect, abuse, or emotional unavailability—the child's developing mind creates explanations that preserve the attachment relationship while making sense of painful experiences.

The process resembles a child trying to solve a puzzle with missing pieces. Unable to comprehend that caregivers might be incapable of meeting their needs, children create internal explanations that place responsibility on themselves. "If mommy doesn't comfort me when I cry, it must be because something is wrong with me," becomes the logical conclusion for a three-year-old mind that depends on mommy for survival.

These early conclusions become **foundational beliefs** that filter all future relationship experiences. A child who develops an abandonment schema doesn't just fear being left alone—they organize their entire personality around preventing abandonment while simultaneously expecting it to happen. This creates the tragic irony we see so often in adults with disconnection schemas: the very behaviors meant to preserve relationships often drive people away.

Neglect operates particularly insidiously because it doesn't involve obvious trauma that adults can easily recognize. A child who experiences sexual abuse may struggle with the aftermath, but they typically understand that something wrong happened to them. A child who experiences emotional neglect may struggle just as much, but they often

51

blame themselves for being "too needy" or "not worthy of attention."

Consider the development of schemas in different family environments. Physical abuse creates mistrust schemas as children learn that people who claim to love them will also hurt them. Emotional abuse creates defectiveness schemas as children internalize critical messages about their fundamental worth. Neglect creates emotional deprivation schemas as children learn that their emotional needs are burdens that others won't willingly meet.

The timing of these experiences matters enormously. Schemas formed during the first three years of life—when attachment patterns are most malleable—often become more deeply ingrained than those formed later. However, significant trauma or ongoing patterns can create schemas at any point during childhood or even early adulthood.

**Recognizing Patterns in Relationships and Self-Perception**

Disconnection and rejection schemas create predictable patterns that show up consistently across different relationships and life situations. Learning to recognize these patterns provides the first step toward changing them.

**Abandonment Schema Patterns** typically involve desperate attempts to prevent real or imagined rejection. People with this schema might check their partner's phone, become extremely upset when friends cancel plans, or choose relationships with unavailable partners who can't truly leave because they were never fully present. The schema creates hypervigilance for signs of rejection while simultaneously interpreting neutral events as evidence of impending abandonment.

Rachel demonstrates classic abandonment patterns. She meets wonderful men who express genuine interest, but as soon as the relationship becomes serious, she begins testing their commitment. She picks fights over small issues, threatens to leave first, or becomes increasingly demanding to see if they'll stay. When partners inevitably become exhausted by this dynamic and withdraw, Rachel feels vindicated—"See, I knew you'd leave eventually"—reinforcing the schema that created the problem.

**Mistrust/Abuse Schema Patterns** involve constant scanning for signs that others will hurt, humiliate, or exploit them. People with this schema often choose relationships that confirm their expectations of betrayal, or they maintain such emotional distance that intimacy becomes impossible. They may be hypervigilant about being taken advantage of financially, emotionally, or sexually, even in relationships with trustworthy people.

**Emotional Deprivation Schema Patterns** create relationships where the person gives constantly but rarely asks for support. They often attract partners who are emotionally unavailable or struggling with their own issues. The schema whispers that asking for emotional support will burden others and ultimately drive them away, creating a self-fulfilling prophecy of emotional starvation.

**Defectiveness Schema Patterns** involve hiding authentic selves while maintaining relationships based on false personas. People with this schema often achieve significant external success while feeling like frauds who will eventually be "found out." They may sabotage relationships when they become too intimate, fearing that being truly known will result in rejection.

**Social Isolation Schema Patterns** create a sense of being fundamentally different from others. People with this schema often feel like outsiders even in groups where they're welcomed and accepted. They may avoid social situations, choose solitary activities, or maintain superficial relationships that don't challenge their belief that they don't belong anywhere.

### Case Studies: Five Detailed Examples of Each Schema in Trauma Survivors

### Abandonment Schema: Jennifer's Story

Jennifer's abandonment schema began forming at age four when her father left the family without warning. One morning he was there reading the newspaper, and the next morning his clothes were gone and her mother was crying in the kitchen. No one explained what happened or helped Jennifer process this sudden loss.

Her mother, overwhelmed by single parenthood and her own abandonment trauma, became emotionally unavailable just when Jennifer needed reassurance most. Jennifer learned that people you love disappear without warning and that expressing needs pushes people away when they're already struggling.

By adolescence, Jennifer had developed a complex abandonment schema that affected every relationship. She chose boyfriends who were emotionally unavailable—men who traveled constantly, were recently divorced, or showed signs of addiction. These relationships felt familiar and manageable because they couldn't trigger her abandonment fears as deeply (you can't be abandoned by someone who was never fully present).

When Jennifer did date someone emotionally available, her schema created chaos. She would call multiple times if he didn't answer immediately, interpret delays in text responses as signs of lost interest, and become devastated when he spent time with friends. Her hypervigilance about abandonment signals created the very rejection she feared.

The turning point came when Jennifer's therapist helped her recognize that her abandonment schema was driving away partners who actually wanted to stay. She learned to identify schema activation—the tight chest, racing thoughts, and urge to check up on her partner—and practiced self-soothing instead of acting on abandonment fears. Most importantly, she began choosing partners based on their emotional availability rather than their familiar unavailability.

**Mistrust/Abuse Schema: Michael's Story**

Michael's mistrust schema developed during years of sexual abuse by his stepfather, which began when he was seven and continued until he was twelve. The abuse involved not just physical violation but psychological manipulation— threats about what would happen if he told anyone, messages that he was special and chosen, and gaslighting that made him doubt his own perceptions.

The schema created by this experience went beyond fear of sexual abuse to include expectation that anyone who got close would eventually exploit or betray him. Michael learned that people who claimed to love him would use that love as a weapon, and that trusting anyone completely was dangerous.

In adult relationships, Michael's mistrust schema created a pattern of choosing partners who confirmed his expectations. He dated people who were financially unstable and might take advantage of his generosity, or those who had histories of infidelity. These relationships felt safer than truly trusting someone because they didn't challenge his core belief that trust inevitably leads to betrayal.

His therapy focused on recognizing the difference between reasonable caution and schema-driven paranoia. Michael learned to identify when his mistrust responses were appropriate (noticing actual red flags in new relationships) versus when they were schema activation (interpreting a partner's privacy needs as evidence of deception). The healing process required gradually practicing trust in small increments while maintaining appropriate boundaries.

**Emotional Deprivation Schema: Sandra's Story**

Sandra grew up with parents who were physically present but emotionally absent. Her father worked sixty-hour weeks and spent evenings watching television, while her mother managed household tasks with efficient detachment. Both parents consistently responded to Sandra's emotional needs with practical solutions—offering food when she was sad, suggesting activities when she was bored, or giving advice when she wanted comfort.

This consistent pattern taught Sandra that emotional needs were problems to be solved rather than experiences to be understood and shared. She learned that expressing feelings made others uncomfortable and that real connection wasn't possible or available to her.

Sandra's adult relationships reflected this early learning. She became the friend everyone turned to for advice and support but rarely shared her own struggles. She chose romantic partners who were dealing with their own crises—addiction, divorce, career problems—so she could focus on helping them rather than risking her own vulnerability.

Her emotional deprivation schema created relationships that felt familiar but left her chronically empty. She gave and gave, hoping that enough caretaking would eventually earn her the emotional connection she craved. But her schema made it impossible to recognize when partners did offer emotional support, filtering their care through the belief that her needs were burdens.

The healing process involved learning to identify her emotional needs and practicing expressing them in small doses. Sandra started by sharing feelings with trusted friends before attempting deeper vulnerability with romantic partners. She discovered that many people actually wanted to support her emotionally but had learned to respect her apparent preference for caretaking over receiving care.

### Defectiveness Schema: Carlos's Story

Carlos's defectiveness schema developed from years of emotional abuse disguised as high expectations. His parents, both successful professionals, consistently communicated that his efforts weren't good enough. An A-minus grade warranted questions about why it wasn't an A-plus. Success in sports led to comparisons with more talented teammates. Any expression of struggle or difficulty was met with disappointment and suggestions that he wasn't trying hard enough.

These experiences taught Carlos that his authentic self—complete with normal human struggles and limitations—was unacceptable. He learned to present a false self that appeared confident and capable while hiding any evidence of the problems and insecurities that might reveal his "true" defective nature.

Carlos became extraordinarily successful professionally, driven by his defectiveness schema's demand for external validation. He worked extreme hours, took on impossible projects, and achieved recognition that temporarily quieted the internal voice insisting he was fooling everyone. But success never felt satisfying because the schema insisted it was based on deception rather than genuine worth.

His relationships suffered because intimacy threatened to expose the flaws he worked so hard to hide. Carlos chose partners who were impressed by his achievements but didn't know him deeply, or he sabotaged relationships when they became too close. The schema convinced him that being truly known would result in inevitable rejection.

Recovery required Carlos to practice radical honesty about his struggles and limitations. He learned to share fears, mistakes, and uncertainties with trusted friends and eventually with romantic partners. The terrifying discovery was that people often felt closer to him when he showed vulnerability rather than pushing him away as his schema predicted.

**Social Isolation Schema: Teresa's Story**

Teresa's social isolation schema began in early childhood when her family moved frequently due to her father's military career. By age ten, she had attended seven different schools and learned that forming close friendships was painful because they always ended. Rather than experience repeated loss, Teresa began keeping emotional distance from peers, telling herself she preferred being alone.

Her family dynamics reinforced this pattern. Her parents, dealing with their own stress from frequent relocations, encouraged Teresa to be independent and self-reliant. They praised her for not complaining about moves and for adapting quickly to new situations. Teresa learned that needing others was a weakness and that being different (the perpetual new kid) was her natural state.

The schema solidified during adolescence when Teresa struggled to connect with peers who had shared histories and established friend groups. She interpreted their exclusion as evidence that she was fundamentally different and would never fit in anywhere. Rather than continue risking rejection, she embraced her outsider status and focused on academic achievement.

As an adult, Teresa maintained the social isolation pattern even in stable environments. She worked in technical fields that required minimal social interaction, lived alone, and maintained superficial friendships that didn't challenge her belief that she was too different for genuine connection. The schema created a self-fulfilling prophecy—her emotional distance convinced others that she wasn't interested in friendship, confirming her belief that she didn't belong.

Healing required Teresa to challenge her assumption that being different meant being unacceptable. She began joining groups based on shared interests rather than trying to fit into existing social circles. Most importantly, she learned that many people actually valued the unique perspective her different experiences provided, rather than seeing her background as a barrier to connection.

**Professional Treatment Protocols for Each Schema**

Schema therapy provides specific treatment protocols for addressing disconnection and rejection schemas, recognizing that each pattern requires different therapeutic approaches while maintaining consistent underlying principles of safety, validation, and gradual exposure to corrective experiences.

**Abandonment Schema Treatment Protocol**

**Phase 1: Recognition and Stabilization**

- Help clients identify abandonment triggers and typical responses

- Develop grounding techniques for managing activation intensity

- Create safety plans for high-risk periods (partner travel, relationship changes)

- Educate about schema development to reduce self-blame

**Phase 2: Cognitive Restructuring**

- Challenge catastrophic predictions about relationship outcomes

- Examine evidence for and against abandonment fears

- Develop balanced thoughts about relationship security and normal fluctuations

- Practice reality testing when schema activation occurs

**Phase 3: Experiential Work**

- Use imagery rescripting to address original abandonment experiences

- Practice expressing needs without desperation or testing behaviors

- Role-play difficult conversations about relationship concerns

- Develop capacity to tolerate uncertainty in relationships

**Phase 4: Behavioral Pattern-Breaking**

- Reduce checking and reassurance-seeking behaviors gradually

- Practice self-soothing instead of immediate contact with partners

- Choose relationships based on actual availability rather than familiar unavailability

- Develop independent activities and friendships to reduce partner dependence

**Mistrust/Abuse Schema Treatment Protocol**

**Phase 1: Safety and Trauma Processing**

- Ensure current safety and address ongoing trauma if present

- Process specific abuse experiences through trauma-focused techniques

- Develop capacity to distinguish past trauma from present relationships
- Create safety protocols for managing trauma activation

## Phase 2: Trust Discrimination

- Learn to assess trustworthiness based on evidence rather than assumptions
- Practice graduated trust-building in low-risk relationships
- Develop skills for setting appropriate boundaries
- Challenge black-and-white thinking about trust and betrayal

## Phase 3: Relationship Skills

- Practice expressing needs and concerns directly rather than through testing
- Learn to recognize and communicate about trust ruptures and repairs
- Develop capacity for appropriate vulnerability in safe relationships
- Address sexual intimacy issues if relevant to abuse history

## Phase 4: Integration and Maintenance

- Maintain awareness of trauma history without letting it control present choices
- Continue practicing trust discrimination skills

- Develop support network of trustworthy relationships

- Create ongoing safety plan for trauma anniversary reactions

**Emotional Deprivation Schema Treatment Protocol**

**Phase 1: Need Recognition**

- Help clients identify emotional needs they've learned to suppress

- Validate the legitimacy of human needs for emotional connection

- Explore family-of-origin messages about emotional expression

- Develop language for different emotional experiences

**Phase 2: Expression Skills**

- Practice expressing emotions and needs in small, manageable doses

- Learn to recognize when others offer emotional support

- Develop capacity to receive care without immediately reciprocating

- Challenge beliefs about burdening others with emotional needs

**Phase 3: Relationship Selection**

- Assess current relationships for emotional availability

- Practice choosing friends and partners who can provide emotional support

- End or modify relationships that only involve caretaking

- Develop skills for creating mutual emotional exchange

**Phase 4: Self-Care Integration**

- Learn to meet some emotional needs through self-care rather than only through others

- Develop internal nurturing voice to supplement external support

- Create ongoing practices for emotional self-awareness and expression

- Maintain boundaries around caretaking to preserve energy for receiving care

**Self-Help Strategies: Recognition Exercises and Coping Techniques**

**Daily Schema Monitoring Exercise**

Keep a brief daily log tracking schema activation episodes. For each occurrence, note:

1. **Trigger situation** - What happened that activated the schema?

2. **Physical sensations** - How did the activation feel in your body?

3. **Automatic thoughts** - What thoughts went through your mind?

4. **Emotional response** - What emotions did you experience?

5. **Behavioral urges** - What did you want to do in response?

6. **Actual behavior** - What did you actually do?

7. **Outcome** - How did the situation resolve?

This monitoring helps you recognize patterns and develop alternative responses over time.

**Grounding Technique for Schema Activation**

Schema activation often feels overwhelming and urgent. This five-step grounding technique helps you return to the present moment:

1. **Notice five things you can see** in your immediate environment

2. **Notice four things you can touch** (texture of your clothes, temperature of air)

3. **Notice three things you can hear** (traffic, air conditioning, your breath)

4. **Notice two things you can smell** (coffee, soap, fresh air)

5. **Notice one thing you can taste** (gum, toothpaste, or take a sip of water)

This technique activates your senses and nervous system to reconnect with present reality rather than schema-driven fears.

### Reality Testing Questions

When schema activation occurs, ask yourself these questions to distinguish between schema-driven fears and actual relationship concerns:

- What concrete evidence supports my concern about this situation?

- What evidence contradicts or complicates my initial interpretation?

- How might someone without my schema history interpret this same situation?

- What would I tell a friend who was experiencing this same concern?

- Are my emotional reactions proportional to the actual event that occurred?

- What's the worst realistic outcome, and how would I handle it?

### Self-Compassion Practice for Schema Healing

Schema healing requires developing a more compassionate internal voice to replace the harsh criticism that often accompanies these patterns. Practice this self-compassion technique daily:

1. **Recognize suffering** - "This is a moment of difficulty" or "I'm experiencing pain right now"

2. **Remember common humanity** - "Struggling with relationships is part of human experience" or "Many people have felt this way"

3. **Offer kindness** - "May I be kind to myself in this moment" or "May I give myself the compassion I need"

This practice gradually builds an internal nurturing voice that can comfort you during schema activation without requiring external validation.

## The Path Forward

Disconnection and rejection schemas represent some of the most painful patterns humans can develop—they attack our fundamental need for love and belonging. Yet understanding these patterns provides genuine hope for healing wounds that may have felt permanent for decades.

The five schemas we've explored—abandonment, mistrust/abuse, emotional deprivation, defectiveness, and social isolation—all share a common theme: they developed to protect you from experiencing relationship pain by predicting and controlling it. The tragic irony is that these protective strategies often create the very rejection they were designed to prevent.

Recovery doesn't require eliminating these schemas entirely—they became part of your survival system for good reasons. Instead, healing involves reducing their intensity and developing new responses that serve your current life rather than your childhood survival needs. The same intelligence that developed these protective patterns can learn to recognize when they're activated and choose different responses.

Most importantly, healing from disconnection and rejection schemas happens in relationship. While individual therapy provides essential support, the real healing occurs through experiencing relationships that don't confirm your schema predictions—friends who don't abandon you when you express needs, partners who remain trustworthy over time, and communities that accept your authentic self rather than demanding perfection.

The next part of your journey involves examining how trauma affects your sense of personal power and independence. Impaired autonomy schemas create different but equally challenging patterns that deserve the same compassionate understanding and practical intervention.

**Essential Takeaways from Disconnection and Rejection Patterns**

- These schemas develop when basic needs for safety and connection go unmet during childhood

- Each schema creates predictable relationship patterns that often confirm their original predictions

- Recognition of schema activation provides the first step toward creating different responses

- Professional treatment follows specific phases addressing safety, cognition, emotion, and behavior

- Self-help strategies can supplement professional treatment but rarely provide complete healing alone

- Recovery happens through experiencing relationships that don't confirm schema predictions

- Healing involves reducing schema intensity rather than complete elimination of protective patterns

# Chapter 5: Impaired Autonomy and Performance Schemas

The irony wasn't lost on me as Elena sat in my office describing her latest panic attack—triggered by her boss suggesting she handle a project independently. Here was a thirty-two-year-old woman with two graduate degrees, fluent in three languages, who had traveled extensively throughout Europe and Asia. Yet the thought of completing a work project without constant supervision sent her into a spiral of terror and self-doubt.

Elena's story illuminates the particular cruelty of impaired autonomy schemas. Unlike disconnection schemas that primarily affect relationships, these patterns attack our fundamental sense of competence and independence. They convince us that we're incapable of handling normal life challenges, creating a prison of learned helplessness that can persist even in the face of objective evidence of our capabilities.

The four schemas in this domain—dependence, vulnerability to harm, enmeshment, and failure—develop when children's natural drive toward independence gets discouraged, overwhelmed, or distorted. Sometimes this happens through overprotection that communicates danger at every turn. Other times it results from premature demands for independence without adequate support. Both extremes can create lasting patterns that interfere with healthy autonomy development.

**Overprotection and Trauma's Impact on Independence**

Children possess an innate drive toward mastery and independence that emerges naturally through play, exploration, and age-appropriate challenges. This developmental process requires a delicate balance— enough safety to feel secure while attempting new skills, combined with enough freedom to experience natural consequences and build confidence through success.

Trauma disrupts this balance in multiple ways. **Direct trauma** (abuse, witnessing violence, experiencing accidents) can create lasting fearfulness that makes normal independence feel dangerous. **Indirect trauma** (having anxious parents, living in dangerous neighborhoods, experiencing family instability) can teach children that the world is fundamentally unsafe and that independence increases vulnerability.

But overprotection often creates autonomy problems even without obvious trauma. Parents who've experienced their own trauma or loss may become hypervigilant about their children's safety, inadvertently communicating that normal life activities are dangerous. Children receiving these messages learn to doubt their own competence and to rely on others for assessment of risk and capability.

Consider the difference between healthy protection and autonomy-undermining overprotection. Healthy protection might involve teaching a child to look both ways before crossing streets while allowing them to walk to school with friends. Overprotection might involve driving the child to school daily through high school while constantly warning about traffic dangers, stranger danger, and the multiple ways they could be hurt walking alone.

The overprotected child receives the unintended message that they can't assess or handle normal risks independently. This creates a dependence schema where the person genuinely believes they need others to navigate challenges that most people handle routinely.

**When Safety Becomes a Prison**

Family systems that prioritize safety above growth often create environments where children never learn to tolerate normal levels of uncertainty or challenge. These families may have legitimate reasons for their caution—perhaps they've experienced trauma, loss, or live in genuinely dangerous circumstances. However, the child's developing mind can't distinguish between reasonable caution and excessive fear.

The child learns that feeling anxious or uncertain means danger is present and that the solution is to seek safety through dependence on others or avoidance of challenging situations. This creates a feedback loop where anxiety becomes evidence of actual danger rather than a normal response to new experiences.

Sarah's family exemplifies this pattern. Her mother had survived a childhood marked by neglect and unpredictable caregivers. Determined to provide the safety she never experienced, Sarah's mother created an environment where every potential risk was discussed, planned for, and usually avoided. Family activities were limited to familiar, controllable situations. School struggles were immediately solved by parental intervention rather than allowing Sarah to develop problem-solving skills.

While Sarah felt loved and protected, she never learned to trust her own judgment or tolerate uncertainty. By adulthood, she felt incapable of making decisions without extensive consultation with family members. Job interviews terrified her because she couldn't predict or control the outcome. Dating felt impossible because relationships involved too many unknowns.

The safety that protected Sarah in childhood became a prison in adulthood. Her dependence schema convinced her that independent decision-making was dangerous, even when rational analysis suggested otherwise.

**Case Study: Elena's Struggle with Learned Helplessness**

Elena's impaired autonomy patterns began developing in early childhood through a combination of family dynamics and cultural factors that prioritized protection over independence. Her parents, both professionals who had immigrated to the United States, carried their own trauma from political instability in their home country along with intense pressure to ensure their children's success in their new environment.

This background created a family system where Elena's parents took responsibility for managing most aspects of her life. They chose her activities, helped extensively with homework, made most decisions about her social interactions, and consistently communicated that the outside world was full of dangers and challenges that required careful navigation.

While their intentions were loving, the message Elena internalized was that she couldn't trust her own judgment or handle challenges independently. When problems arose at school or with friends, her parents immediately intervened rather than coaching her through problem-solving. When she expressed interest in activities they considered risky or impractical, they redirected her toward safer alternatives.

Elena excelled academically because her parents provided extensive support and structure. However, she never developed confidence in her own decision-making abilities or learned to tolerate the uncertainty that comes with independent choices. Her achievements felt more like collaborative efforts than personal accomplishments.

The pattern intensified during college when Elena struggled with the freedom and responsibility of independent living. While other students adapted to managing their own schedules, social lives, and academic responsibilities, Elena felt overwhelmed and constantly called home for guidance. She changed majors multiple times, not because of lack of interest, but because each choice felt too permanent and consequential to make alone.

Her dependence schema created a self-perpetuating cycle. The more she relied on others for decisions, the less confidence she developed in her own judgment. The less confidence she had, the more dangerous independent choices felt. By the time she entered the workforce, Elena had convinced herself that she was fundamentally incapable of handling normal adult responsibilities without constant guidance.

The turning point came during a therapy session where Elena realized that her panic about independent work projects stemmed not from actual incompetence, but from beliefs about her capabilities that no longer matched reality. She had successfully completed graduate school, managed international travel, and handled numerous personal challenges. Yet her dependence schema filtered these experiences through the lens of luck or help from others rather than recognizing her own competence.

Recovery required Elena to practice making decisions in low-risk situations while learning to tolerate the anxiety that accompanied independent choice-making. She started with small decisions—choosing restaurants, planning weekend activities, selecting books to read—and gradually worked up to larger choices about career direction and relationships.

Most importantly, Elena learned to distinguish between the voice of her dependence schema ("You can't handle this; you need help") and the voice of genuine wisdom ("This situation actually does require consultation or support"). The schema voice felt panicked and absolute, while genuine wisdom felt calm and discriminating.

**Building Healthy Autonomy After Trauma**

Healthy autonomy develops through gradual exposure to age-appropriate challenges combined with reliable support when genuine difficulties arise. For people with impaired autonomy schemas, this developmental process needs to happen consciously in adulthood, often requiring therapeutic support to create the safety and structure necessary for growth.

The process begins with **recognizing the difference between schema-driven fears and legitimate concerns**. Schema fears tend to be global ("I can't handle anything difficult"), absolute ("If I make the wrong choice, everything will be ruined"), and disproportionate to actual risk ("Choosing the wrong job will destroy my life"). Legitimate concerns are specific ("I need more information about this particular decision"), proportionate ("This choice has some risks I should consider"), and solvable ("I can gather more information or seek consultation").

**Building distress tolerance** becomes essential because autonomy development inevitably involves uncertainty and occasional mistakes. People with impaired autonomy schemas often can't distinguish between discomfort and danger, leading them to seek safety whenever they feel anxious or uncertain. Learning that discomfort is a normal part of growth rather than a signal to retreat requires both conceptual understanding and practical experience.

**Developing decision-making skills** involves learning systematic approaches to choices rather than relying on intuition or others' opinions. This might include gathering relevant information, considering multiple options, weighing pros and cons, making time-limited decisions, and accepting that most choices can be adjusted if they don't work out as expected.

**Creating appropriate support systems** means distinguishing between dependency and healthy interdependence. Everyone needs input and support for major decisions, but people with autonomy schemas often can't tell the difference between normal consultation and excessive reliance on others. Healthy autonomy includes knowing when to seek support and how to use input without surrendering personal responsibility.

**Professional Protocol: Graduated Exposure and Empowerment Strategies**

Schema therapy approaches impaired autonomy patterns through systematic exposure to independence-building experiences, always balanced with adequate support to prevent overwhelming anxiety that could reinforce dependence patterns.

**Phase 1: Assessment and Psychoeducation**

**Identifying Schema Triggers** Therapists help clients recognize specific situations that activate their autonomy schemas. Common triggers include:

- Making decisions without consultation

- Handling problems independently

- Facing unfamiliar challenges

- Taking responsibility for outcomes

- Managing uncertainty or unpredictability

**Understanding Schema Development** Clients explore how their autonomy patterns developed, often discovering that their "incompetence" beliefs formed in environments where independence was either dangerous or discouraged. This understanding reduces self-blame and creates hope for change.

**Distinguishing Schemas from Reality** Therapists help clients recognize the difference between schema-driven fears and actual limitations or risks. This often involves reviewing evidence of past competence that the schema has discounted or attributed to external factors.

**Phase 2: Cognitive Restructuring**

**Challenging Catastrophic Predictions** Autonomy schemas often predict terrible outcomes from independent action. Cognitive work helps clients examine evidence for these predictions and develop more realistic assessments of risk and consequence.

**Building Self-Efficacy Beliefs** Therapists guide clients in recognizing their existing competencies and reframing past successes as evidence of capability rather than luck or help from others.

**Developing Growth Mindset** Clients learn to view mistakes and struggles as normal parts of learning rather than evidence of fundamental incompetence.

**Phase 3: Graduated Behavioral Experiments**

**Low-Risk Independence Practice** Clients begin practicing independent decision-making and problem-solving in situations with minimal consequences. This might include:

- Choosing restaurants or entertainment without consultation

- Handling minor household problems independently

- Making small purchases based on personal preference

- Planning short trips or outings alone

**Medium-Risk Challenges** As confidence builds, clients tackle more significant challenges:

- Making work decisions within their area of responsibility

- Handling conflict situations without immediate help

- Managing health or financial decisions independently

- Pursuing personal interests despite others' concerns

**High-Risk Autonomy Building** Eventually, clients practice independence in major life areas:

- Career changes or job searches

- Relationship decisions including marriage or breakups

- Major financial choices like home purchases

- Geographic moves or lifestyle changes

### Phase 4: Relapse Prevention and Integration

**Recognizing Schema Activation** Clients learn to identify when autonomy schemas are being triggered so they can respond consciously rather than automatically reverting to dependence patterns.

**Maintaining Support Systems** Healthy autonomy includes knowing when and how to seek appropriate support. Clients learn to distinguish between schema-driven dependency and legitimate needs for consultation or help.

**Ongoing Skill Development** Autonomy building continues throughout life as new challenges arise. Clients develop frameworks for approaching unfamiliar situations with confidence rather than automatic assumption of incompetence.

### Practical Independence-Building Exercises

### The Daily Decision Log

For one week, keep track of every decision you make during the day, no matter how small. Include:

- What decision you faced

- How you made the choice

- Any consultation you sought

- How you felt about the outcome

This exercise helps you recognize how many decisions you already make successfully while identifying patterns of excessive consultation or avoidance.

**The Competence Inventory**

Create a detailed list of things you can do independently, organized by category:

**Practical Skills:** Cooking, driving, using technology, managing money, household maintenance **Social Skills:** Making conversation, handling conflict, maintaining friendships, dating **Work Skills:** Job tasks, project management, problem-solving, learning new systems **Personal Management:** Healthcare decisions, time management, emotional regulation, self-care

Review this list whenever your dependence schema suggests you're incapable of handling challenges.

**The Graduated Challenge Exercise**

Choose one area where you'd like to build more independence. Create a ladder of challenges from easiest to most difficult:

**Example: Building Work Independence**

1. Make a minor work decision without asking for input

2. Handle a routine problem independently

3. Volunteer for a project you can manage alone

4. Lead a small team or initiative

5. Make a significant decision within your authority

6. Take on a stretch assignment that requires new learning

Practice each level until it feels manageable before moving to the next challenge.

**The Anxiety Tolerance Practice**

Since autonomy building often triggers anxiety, practice tolerating uncomfortable feelings without immediately seeking safety:

1. **Notice anxiety arising** during independent activities

2. **Name the feeling** ("I'm feeling anxious about this decision")

3. **Remind yourself** ("Anxiety doesn't mean danger; it means I'm growing")

4. **Use grounding techniques** (deep breathing, body awareness)

5. **Continue the activity** despite the discomfort

6. **Celebrate the practice** regardless of the outcome

This builds capacity to act independently even when feeling uncertain or uncomfortable.

**Distinguishing Between Healthy Caution and Schema-Driven Fear**

One of the most challenging aspects of healing autonomy schemas involves learning when caution is appropriate versus when fear is schema-driven. This discrimination becomes essential for making sound decisions about risk and independence.

**Schema-driven fears** typically have these characteristics:

- They feel overwhelming and paralyzing

- They predict catastrophic outcomes from normal risks

- They generalize across multiple situations

- They don't respond to evidence or reassurance

- They create avoidance of normal life activities

- They persist even when you have relevant competence or experience

**Healthy caution** typically involves:

- Proportionate concern about actual risks

- Specific worry about particular situations

- Responsiveness to information and evidence

- Motivation to gather more data or seek appropriate consultation

- Acceptance of uncertainty while still taking action

- Recognition of your competence while acknowledging limitations

Learning this distinction allows you to honor genuine concerns while not letting schema fears control your choices. It's the difference between avoiding all challenging decisions (schema fear) and gathering information before making important choices (healthy caution).

**Breaking Free from Internal Barriers**

Impaired autonomy schemas represent some of the most limiting patterns humans can develop because they attack our sense of personal agency and competence. They convince us that we're fundamentally incapable of handling what most people manage routinely, creating internal barriers that can be more restrictive than any external obstacle.

Yet these patterns developed for protective reasons. The child who learned to depend on others for decision-making often did so in environments where independence felt dangerous or was actively discouraged. The person who fears failure may have experienced criticism or abandonment when struggling with challenges. Understanding these origins helps transform self-criticism into self-compassion.

Recovery from autonomy schemas requires courage—the willingness to feel anxious and uncertain while building competence through direct experience. This process can't be rushed or forced, but it also can't wait until you feel completely confident. Confidence comes from action, not the other way around.

The beautiful paradox of autonomy building is that the very act of tolerating uncertainty and taking independent action gradually reduces the schema's power. Each small success provides evidence that contradicts the schema's predictions. Each challenge you handle independently strengthens your trust in your own capabilities.

Most importantly, building healthy autonomy doesn't mean isolation or rejection of all support. Mature independence includes knowing when to seek consultation, how to collaborate effectively, and when to accept help gracefully. The goal isn't complete self-reliance but rather confidence in your ability to handle life's challenges while maintaining meaningful connections with others.

**Essential Takeaways from Autonomy and Performance Patterns**

- These schemas develop when children's natural drive toward independence gets discouraged or overwhelmed

- Overprotection can create dependency patterns even in loving families without obvious trauma

- Recovery requires graduated exposure to independence-building experiences with adequate support

- Distinguishing between schema fears and legitimate caution becomes essential for sound decision-making

- Healthy autonomy includes knowing when to seek appropriate support rather than complete self-reliance

- Confidence builds through action rather than waiting to feel ready before taking independent steps

- The goal is developing trust in your capability while maintaining meaningful connections with others

# Chapter 6: Impaired Limits Schemas

David's transformation shocked everyone who knew him, including David himself. For thirty-eight years, he had been the person everyone could count on—the friend who dropped everything to help with moves, the employee who worked weekends without complaint, the son who managed his aging parents' affairs while his siblings lived their own lives. He wore his selflessness like a badge of honor, genuinely believing that his worth depended on his willingness to sacrifice for others.

Then came the day his teenage daughter asked why he never seemed to have opinions about anything important to him. "You always ask what we want, Dad. But what do you want?" The question hit David like a physical blow because he realized he had no idea how to answer it. Somewhere along the way, he had lost touch with his own desires, needs, and boundaries so completely that he no longer knew where others ended and he began.

David's story illustrates the complex nature of impaired limits schemas—patterns that can look like admirable selflessness from the outside while creating internal chaos and relationship dysfunction underneath. The two schemas in this domain, entitlement and insufficient self-control, might seem contradictory at first glance, but they both reflect problems with healthy boundary development and emotional regulation.

### How Trauma Can Lead to Both Under-Control and Over-Control

Trauma affects limit-setting and self-control in paradoxical ways, sometimes creating patterns that swing between extremes of rigidity and chaos. Understanding these patterns requires recognizing that healthy limits involve a flexible balance—knowing when to assert your needs and when to consider others, when to control impulses and when to express them appropriately.

**Under-control patterns** often develop when children grow up without consistent limits or consequences. This might happen in families struggling with addiction, mental illness, or trauma where parents can't provide stable structure. Children in these environments may never learn to delay gratification, consider consequences, or respect others' boundaries because no one taught them these skills.

But under-control can also develop from trauma that creates intense emotional reactivity. When a child's nervous system becomes dysregulated by abuse, neglect, or chaotic family dynamics, they may struggle with impulse control not because of lack of limits, but because their emotional system is overwhelmed. The brain's capacity for self-regulation gets disrupted by chronic stress and trauma exposure.

**Over-control patterns** frequently emerge as responses to chaotic or dangerous environments. The child who develops excessive self-control may be trying to prevent abuse, maintain family stability, or earn love through perfect behavior. This strategy can become so automatic that the person loses touch with their authentic impulses and needs.

Consider Maria's development of insufficient self-control following childhood sexual abuse. The trauma created emotional dysregulation that made normal impulse control extremely difficult. When triggered by stress or relationship conflicts, Maria would experience overwhelming rage,

86

engage in self-destructive behaviors, or make impulsive decisions that damaged her relationships and career.

On the surface, Maria's behavior looked like selfishness or lack of consideration for others. But underneath, her insufficient self-control represented trauma responses that she had never learned to manage effectively. The shame about her lack of control then created additional trauma, perpetuating the cycle.

Contrast this with James's development of over-control in response to an alcoholic father whose unpredictable rages terrified the family. James learned that any expression of his own needs, emotions, or preferences could trigger his father's anger, potentially putting himself and his mother at risk. He developed such rigid self-control that by adulthood, he had almost no awareness of his own wants and feelings.

James appeared highly functional and considerate, but his over-control created problems in intimate relationships where emotional authenticity and mutual exchange were necessary. His pattern looked like virtue but actually represented trauma-based suppression of normal human needs and emotions.

**Boundary Issues in Trauma Survivors**

Trauma fundamentally disrupts the development of healthy boundaries—the psychological and emotional limits that define where you end and others begin. Children who experience trauma often learn boundary patterns that prioritize survival over healthy relationship dynamics.

**Boundary violation** teaches children that their physical and emotional limits don't matter or will be ignored. They may learn to accommodate others' needs automatically while suppressing their own, creating patterns that persist long after the original danger has passed.

**Boundary confusion** occurs when children receive inconsistent messages about limits. A parent might be loving and respectful one day, then intrusive and demanding the next, leaving the child unable to predict what boundaries will be honored.

**Boundary rigidity** can develop when children decide that the safest strategy is to trust no one and need nothing from others. These children may grow into adults who appear independent but are actually isolated by their inability to form genuine connections.

**Boundary permeability** creates patterns where the person can't distinguish between their emotions and others', often becoming overwhelmed by others' feelings while losing touch with their own experiences.

Lisa's boundary development illustrates these complexities. Growing up with a mother who struggled with severe depression, Lisa learned to monitor her mother's emotional state constantly and adjust her own behavior to maintain family stability. She became so attuned to others' needs that she lost awareness of her own feelings and preferences.

As an adult, Lisa attracted people who needed extensive emotional support while avoiding those who might expect mutual exchange. Her relationships felt familiar but ultimately unsatisfying because they replicated the childhood pattern of caretaking without receiving care.

The challenge for Lisa involved learning to recognize her own emotional and physical limits while maintaining her natural compassion for others. This required developing what trauma specialists call "differentiation"—the ability to care about others without taking responsibility for their emotional well-being.

## Case Study: David's Journey from Victim to Accountability

David's journey toward healthy boundaries began with recognizing how his pattern of compulsive caretaking actually represented a form of control rather than genuine generosity. While he appeared selfless, his behavior often prevented others from developing their own problem-solving skills and created relationships based on dependence rather than mutual respect.

**Childhood Pattern Development** David grew up as the oldest child in a family where his mother struggled with chronic anxiety and his father worked excessive hours to avoid emotional demands at home. David discovered early that he could reduce family tension by anticipating and meeting everyone's needs before they expressed them.

This strategy earned him praise as a "helpful" and "mature" child, but it also taught him that his worth depended on his usefulness to others. David learned to scan constantly for others' needs while suppressing his own, creating a pattern that felt virtuous but was actually driven by fear of rejection and abandonment.

**Adult Pattern Recognition** By his late thirties, David's caretaking pattern had created several problems. His marriage felt more like a parent-child relationship where he handled most responsibilities while his wife remained dependent on his management. His children appreciated his help but never learned to handle normal challenges independently. His friendships were one-sided relationships where others came to him for support but rarely offered reciprocal care.

Most concerning, David had developed physical symptoms—chronic headaches, digestive problems, and insomnia—that his doctor attributed to stress. David couldn't understand why he felt so overwhelmed when he was "just helping people," not recognizing that his compulsive caretaking represented a form of self-neglect that was taking a serious toll.

**The Turning Point** David's wake-up call came during a family crisis when his elderly father was hospitalized. While David immediately took charge of managing medical decisions, coordinating care, and supporting family members, his siblings remained passive, expecting him to handle everything as usual.

The moment of clarity came when David realized he felt resentful and angry about carrying all the responsibility, but he had never asked for help or set any limits on what he would manage. His "helpful" behavior had actually trained his family to depend on him while preventing them from taking appropriate responsibility.

**Learning Healthy Boundaries** David's therapy focused on helping him distinguish between genuine helpfulness and compulsive caretaking. He learned to recognize the difference between others' requests for support and his automatic assumption of responsibility for their problems.

The process began with small boundary-setting exercises. Instead of immediately offering solutions when friends shared problems, David practiced listening and asking what kind of support they wanted. Instead of managing his wife's schedule and responsibilities, he began letting her handle her own commitments while offering assistance only when specifically requested.

Initially, these changes felt uncomfortable and selfish to David. His schema whispered that he was being uncaring and that people would reject him if he wasn't constantly helpful. However, David discovered that most people actually appreciated his increased respect for their autonomy and competence.

**Integration and Growth** Six months into his boundary work, David noticed several significant changes. His physical symptoms had decreased dramatically as his stress levels dropped. His relationships had become more mutual, with others offering support to him as well as receiving it. Most surprisingly, his help felt more meaningful to others because it came from choice rather than compulsion.

David learned that healthy boundaries don't eliminate generosity—they make generosity more sustainable and authentic. By taking care of his own needs and setting appropriate limits, he had more energy and presence to offer when others genuinely needed support.

The most profound change was David's relationship with his own needs and preferences. After years of focusing exclusively on others, he began rediscovering his interests, opinions, and desires. This felt uncomfortable initially, but gradually David experienced the relief of being authentic rather than constantly performing helpfulness.

### Teaching Healthy Boundaries and Self-Regulation

Developing healthy limits requires learning skills that many trauma survivors missed during childhood. These skills can be developed at any age, but they require conscious practice and often benefit from therapeutic support, especially when trauma has created complex patterns around control and boundaries.

### Understanding Different Types of Boundaries

**Physical boundaries** involve your comfort with touch, personal space, and physical intimacy. Healthy physical boundaries include saying no to unwanted touch, asking for space when needed, and expressing preferences about physical closeness.

**Emotional boundaries** protect your emotional well-being by limiting how much responsibility you take for others' feelings while maintaining appropriate care and compassion. This includes not automatically absorbing others' emotions as your own and not feeling responsible for managing others' emotional states.

**Mental boundaries** involve your right to your own thoughts, opinions, and beliefs. Healthy mental boundaries include expressing disagreement respectfully, not automatically adopting others' viewpoints to maintain harmony, and recognizing that you don't need others' approval for your perspectives.

**Time and energy boundaries** protect your resources by ensuring that you have adequate time and energy for your own needs and priorities. This includes saying no to requests that would overextend you and prioritizing activities that support your well-being.

**Material boundaries** involve your comfort with lending, borrowing, and sharing possessions or money. Healthy material boundaries include making conscious choices about financial support and not automatically sharing resources to avoid conflict.

### Developing Emotional Regulation Skills

Trauma often disrupts the natural development of emotional regulation—the ability to experience emotions without being overwhelmed by them and to express feelings in ways that are appropriate to the situation.

**Emotional awareness** forms the foundation of regulation. This involves learning to identify what you're feeling in the moment rather than automatically suppressing or acting on emotions. Many trauma survivors developed such effective emotional suppression that they struggle to recognize their feelings until they become overwhelming.

**Distress tolerance** involves learning to experience uncomfortable emotions without immediately trying to escape or change them. This might include staying present with anxiety, sadness, or anger long enough to understand what the emotions are trying to communicate.

**Expression skills** help you communicate emotions in ways that are clear and appropriate rather than suppressed or explosively released. This includes using "I" statements, expressing needs directly, and timing emotional conversations appropriately.

**Self-soothing techniques** provide ways to comfort yourself during emotional distress without relying exclusively on others or engaging in harmful behaviors. This might include breathing exercises, physical movement, creative expression, or mindfulness practices.

**Intervention Guide: Limit-Setting Exercises and Techniques**

**The Boundary Awareness Exercise**

For one week, pay attention to moments when you feel uncomfortable, resentful, or overwhelmed in relationships. Notice:

- What was happening when the feeling arose?

- What boundary might have been crossed or needed?

- How did you respond in the moment?

- What would a healthy boundary have looked like in that situation?

This exercise helps you recognize when boundaries are needed rather than automatically accommodating others' requests or demands.

**The Graduated "No" Practice**

Many trauma survivors struggle with saying no directly because they learned that refusal led to conflict or rejection. Practice saying no in increasingly challenging situations:

**Level 1:** Decline invitations to activities you don't enjoy
**Level 2:** Say no to requests for help when you're already overextended
**Level 3:** Disagree with opinions you don't share **Level 4:** Set limits on behavior that makes you uncomfortable **Level 5:** End conversations or interactions that feel harmful

Start with situations that feel manageable and gradually work toward more challenging boundary-setting opportunities.

## The Needs Identification Exercise

Since trauma survivors often lose touch with their own needs while focusing on others, practice identifying and expressing your preferences:

**Daily needs:** What do you need for physical comfort, emotional well-being, and practical functioning each day?

**Relationship needs:** What do you need to feel valued, respected, and connected in your relationships?

**Work needs:** What do you need to feel engaged, competent, and fairly treated in your professional life?

**Personal growth needs:** What do you need to continue learning, developing, and expressing your authentic self?

Practice expressing these needs in small, low-risk situations before attempting to communicate about major relationship or life issues.

## The Emotional Regulation Toolbox

Develop a collection of techniques for managing emotional intensity that you can use in different situations:

**For anxiety:** Deep breathing, progressive muscle relaxation, grounding exercises using your five senses

**For anger:** Physical movement, journaling, talking to a trusted friend, taking a temporary break from the situation

**For sadness:** Allowing tears, seeking comfort from supportive people, engaging in nurturing self-care activities

**For overwhelm:** Simplifying your environment, reducing stimulation, focusing on one task at a time

**For emotional numbness:** Gentle movement, listening to music, engaging in creative activities, spending time in nature

Practice these techniques when you're calm so they're available during times of emotional distress.

### The Values Clarification Process

Trauma can disconnect you from your authentic values and priorities. Spend time identifying what matters most to you across different life areas:

**Relationships:** What qualities do you value in friendships and partnerships? How do you want to treat others and be treated?

**Work:** What kind of contribution do you want to make? What work environment supports your well-being?

**Personal growth:** What aspects of yourself do you want to develop? What experiences do you want to have?

**Community:** How do you want to contribute to your family, community, or causes you care about?

Use these values as guides for making decisions and setting boundaries rather than automatically accommodating others' expectations.

### The Integration of Control and Freedom

Healthy limits schemas represent a sophisticated balance between self-control and spontaneous expression, between consideration for others and attention to your own needs.

This balance can't be achieved through rules or rigid formulas—it requires developing internal wisdom that can assess each situation and respond appropriately.

The goal isn't perfect boundary-setting or flawless emotional regulation. Instead, it's developing the capacity to recognize when limits are needed and the courage to set them even when it feels uncomfortable. It's learning to experience emotions without being controlled by them while still honoring what your feelings are trying to tell you.

For trauma survivors, developing healthy limits often feels selfish or dangerous initially because their schemas were formed in environments where self-assertion led to negative consequences. The healing process requires gradually discovering that healthy boundaries actually improve relationships by creating space for authentic connection rather than forced compliance.

Most importantly, healing from impaired limits schemas involves recognizing that your needs, feelings, and preferences matter as much as others'. This doesn't mean becoming self-centered or inconsiderate—it means including yourself in the circle of people you treat with respect and compassion.

The journey toward healthy limits is ultimately a journey toward authentic selfhood. As you learn to honor your own boundaries while respecting others', you create space for relationships based on choice rather than obligation, mutual respect rather than caretaking, and genuine care rather than fear-based compliance.

## Core Principles for Developing Healthy Limits

- Boundaries protect relationships by preventing resentment and promoting authenticity

- Saying no to some requests allows you to say yes more genuinely to others

- Emotional regulation involves experiencing feelings without being controlled by them

- Healthy limits include both self-assertion and consideration for others

- Values provide guidance for boundary decisions rather than automatic accommodation of others' expectations

- Practice in low-risk situations builds capacity for setting limits in more challenging circumstances

- The goal is balance between self-care and care for others, not elimination of either

# Chapter 7: Other-Directedness Schemas

Maria could pinpoint the exact moment her life began to unravel, though it would take months of therapy to understand why such a small incident had triggered such a massive crisis. She was standing in line at a coffee shop when the barista asked what she'd like to order. For reasons she couldn't explain, Maria's mind went completely blank. She couldn't remember what kind of coffee she usually ordered, what she was in the mood for, or even what she generally liked. The simple question "What would you like?" felt impossible to answer because Maria realized she had no idea what she actually wanted.

At thirty-one, Maria had built a life that looked successful from the outside—a stable relationship, a respected career in social work, close friendships, and a reputation as someone people could always count on for support and advice. Yet standing in that coffee shop, she confronted the terrifying reality that she had no idea who she actually was underneath all the roles she played for others.

Maria's experience illuminates the particular suffering created by other-directedness schemas—patterns that can look like virtue from the outside while slowly eroding the person's sense of authentic self. The three schemas in this domain—subjugation, self-sacrifice, and approval-seeking— all involve organizing your life around others' needs, expectations, and emotional states while losing touch with your own inner experience.

**The People-Pleasing Trauma Response**

People-pleasing often gets dismissed as a minor personality quirk or an admirable desire to help others. But for trauma survivors, people-pleasing frequently represents a sophisticated survival strategy that developed in environments where the child's safety or emotional security depended on managing others' emotional states.

**Fawn response** represents one of the four primary trauma responses (alongside fight, flight, and freeze) and involves attempting to appease or please potential threats to maintain safety. Children who develop fawn responses often do so in families where conflict is dangerous, emotional expression leads to punishment, or love feels conditional on good behavior.

The fawn response becomes problematic when it persists into adulthood and gets applied to relationships that don't actually threaten the person's safety. The adult who learned to monitor and manage a parent's anger to prevent abuse may continue this pattern with bosses, partners, and friends who have no intention of causing harm.

Consider Anna's development of people-pleasing patterns in response to her mother's untreated mental illness. Anna's mother experienced dramatic mood swings that could shift from loving warmth to explosive rage without warning. Anna learned that she could sometimes prevent these episodes by being exceptionally good—anticipating her mother's needs, avoiding any behavior that might be perceived as demanding, and becoming a source of comfort when her mother felt distressed.

This strategy worked well enough to help Anna survive a chaotic childhood, but it created lasting patterns that interfered with adult relationships. Anna became so skilled at reading and responding to others' emotional states that she lost touch with her own feelings and needs. She attracted people who appreciated her caretaking abilities but struggled to form relationships based on mutual exchange rather than one-sided giving.

## When Survival Depends on Others' Approval

Children who develop other-directedness schemas often grow up in environments where love, safety, or basic needs feel conditional on their behavior. These children learn that their worth depends on external validation rather than internal sense of self, creating patterns that persist long after the original circumstances change.

**Conditional love** teaches children that affection and care depend on meeting others' expectations rather than being loved for who they are. Children receiving conditional love may become hypervigilant about others' approval while losing touch with their authentic selves.

**Emotional parentification** occurs when children become responsible for managing adults' emotional needs. These children may feel valued for their caretaking abilities but never experience being cared for themselves, creating patterns of compulsive giving combined with difficulty receiving support.

**Performance-based worth** develops in families where children's value seems to depend on achievements, good behavior, or fulfilling specific roles. These children may become successful but feel like imposters who are constantly at risk of being discovered as inadequate.

Rachel's story illustrates how approval-seeking patterns develop in response to emotionally unstable family environments. Rachel's father struggled with alcohol addiction, creating unpredictable family dynamics where his mood determined everyone else's emotional state. Rachel learned that she could sometimes improve family atmosphere by being entertaining, achieving academically, or helping manage household responsibilities.

While Rachel's efforts sometimes helped, they also taught her that her worth depended on her ability to make others happy. She became a master at reading social dynamics and adjusting her behavior to maintain harmony, but she lost touch with her own preferences, opinions, and emotional needs.

As an adult, Rachel continued seeking approval through achievement and caretaking. She chose a demanding career in public relations where success depended on managing others' perceptions, maintained friendships that required extensive emotional support, and chose romantic partners who needed fixing rather than those who could offer mutual partnership.

The exhaustion and resentment that eventually developed surprised Rachel because she genuinely enjoyed helping others and took pride in her ability to make people happy. She couldn't understand why activities that felt meaningful also left her feeling empty and disconnected from herself.

**Case Study: Maria's Pattern of Self-Abandonment**

Maria's other-directedness patterns began forming in early childhood through a combination of family dynamics that made her own needs feel dangerous and burdensome. Her parents, both hardworking immigrants, carried significant stress from financial pressures and cultural adaptation while trying to provide opportunities for their children.

**Early Pattern Development** Maria's parents loved their children deeply but had little emotional bandwidth for normal childhood needs like comfort during distress, patience with mistakes, or enthusiasm for childish interests. Maria learned early that expressing needs created additional stress for parents who were already overwhelmed.

Instead of learning that her needs mattered, Maria developed strategies for minimizing the burden she placed on others. She became an exceptionally "easy" child who rarely complained, helped with household tasks, and focused on achieving academically to make her parents proud rather than expressing typical childhood emotions or requests for attention.

This pattern earned Maria praise and affection, but it also taught her that love required constant vigilance about others' emotional capacity and needs. She learned to scan constantly for signs that others were stressed, unhappy, or burdened, adjusting her behavior to maintain harmony and avoid creating additional problems.

**Adolescent Reinforcement** During adolescence, Maria's pattern intensified as she became the family mediator during conflicts between parents and siblings. Her ability to understand multiple perspectives and find compromise solutions made her valuable to family functioning, but it also reinforced her role as the person responsible for managing others' emotional well-being.

Maria's romantic relationships followed similar patterns. She was attracted to partners who were dealing with significant challenges—depression, family problems, career struggles—because these relationships felt familiar and allowed her to focus on caretaking rather than risking vulnerability about her own needs.

**Adult Crisis and Recognition** The coffee shop incident that triggered Maria's crisis represented a moment when her self-abandonment pattern became impossible to ignore. Years of focusing exclusively on others' needs had left her so disconnected from her own preferences that she couldn't answer the simplest question about what she wanted.

This realization forced Maria to confront how thoroughly she had abandoned herself in pursuit of others' approval and comfort. She recognized that her reputation as a caring, supportive person was based on a pattern that left no room for her own authentic self-expression.

**Recovery Process** Maria's healing journey involved learning to recognize and honor her own needs while maintaining her natural compassion for others. This required developing what therapists call "differentiation"—the ability to care about others without taking responsibility for their emotional well-being.

The process began with small experiments in self-assertion. Maria practiced expressing preferences about restaurants, activities, and plans rather than automatically accommodating others' choices. She learned to notice her own emotional responses to situations rather than immediately focusing on how others were feeling.

More challenging was learning to set boundaries with people who had become accustomed to her unlimited availability for emotional support. Maria had to practice saying things like "I care about what you're going through, but I don't have the emotional energy to talk about it right now" while managing her own guilt and others' disappointment.

**Integration and Growth** After a year of conscious practice, Maria reported feeling more authentic and energetic in her relationships. She had lost some friendships that were based primarily on her caretaking function, but her remaining relationships had become more mutual and satisfying.

Most significantly, Maria had begun to experience what she called "internal weather"—awareness of her own emotional states, preferences, and needs that existed independently of others' feelings. This internal experience had been so suppressed that rediscovering it felt like meeting herself for the first time.

### Reclaiming Personal Voice and Needs

The process of healing from other-directedness schemas involves learning to recognize, value, and express your authentic self while maintaining healthy consideration for others. This balance requires developing new skills that many people with these schemas missed during childhood.

### Developing Internal Awareness

**Emotional awareness** forms the foundation of authentic self-expression. Many people with other-directedness schemas learned to suppress their emotional responses so thoroughly that they struggle to identify what they're feeling in real time.

Practice checking in with yourself throughout the day by asking: "What am I feeling right now?" Notice physical sensations, energy levels, and emotional responses without immediately trying to change or justify them.

**Preference recognition** involves learning to identify what you like, dislike, want, and don't want across different life areas. Start with low-stakes preferences like food, entertainment, or activities before moving to more significant choices about relationships or career direction.

**Values clarification** helps you understand what matters most to you rather than automatically adopting others' values to maintain harmony. Spend time reflecting on what you find meaningful, important, and worth pursuing independently of others' expectations.

### Building Expression Skills

**"I" statements** provide a framework for expressing feelings and needs without automatically focusing on others' reactions. Practice statements like "I feel overwhelmed when..." or "I need some time to..." rather than "You make me feel..." or "You should..."

**Boundary language** helps you communicate limits clearly and kindly. Learn phrases like "I'm not comfortable with that," "I need to think about it," or "That doesn't work for me" rather than automatically accommodating requests that don't feel right.

**Disagreement skills** allow you to express different opinions without creating conflict or immediately backing down. Practice expressing disagreement respectfully while maintaining connection: "I see it differently" or "I have a different perspective on that."

## Professional Techniques: Assertiveness Training and Boundary Work

Schema therapy approaches other-directedness patterns through systematic training in self-assertion combined with exploration of the fears and beliefs that maintain people-pleasing patterns.

### Phase 1: Pattern Recognition and Safety Building

**Identifying other-directedness triggers** helps clients recognize situations that automatically activate their people-pleasing responses. Common triggers include:

- Conflict or tension in relationships
- Others expressing disappointment or distress
- Requests for help or support
- Situations requiring personal opinions or preferences
- Social situations where approval feels uncertain

**Understanding schema origins** helps clients recognize how their patterns developed as adaptive responses to specific family dynamics. This reduces self-criticism and creates hope that patterns can change when circumstances no longer require them.

**Building internal safety** involves developing the emotional regulation skills necessary to tolerate others' disappointment or disapproval without automatically reverting to people-pleasing behaviors.

### Phase 2: Cognitive Restructuring

**Challenging approval-seeking beliefs** involves examining thoughts like "I must make everyone happy" or "Conflict means rejection" and developing more balanced perspectives that include your own needs and rights.

**Developing healthy guilt** means learning to distinguish between appropriate guilt (when you've actually harmed someone) and schema-driven guilt (when you've simply prioritized your own needs appropriately).

**Building self-worth independence** involves developing internal sources of validation rather than depending exclusively on others' approval for self-esteem.

### Phase 3: Assertiveness Skill Building

**Graduated assertion practice** begins with low-risk situations and gradually progresses to more challenging assertiveness opportunities:

**Level 1:** Expressing preferences about minor decisions (restaurant choices, entertainment options) **Level 2:** Saying no to requests that would overextend you **Level 3:** Expressing disagreement with others' opinions **Level 4:** Setting boundaries about behavior that makes you uncomfortable **Level 5:** Confronting significant relationship issues directly

**Role-playing difficult conversations** helps clients practice assertiveness skills in the safety of therapy before attempting them in real relationships.

**Managing others' reactions** involves developing strategies for maintaining assertiveness even when others respond with disappointment, anger, or withdrawal.

### Phase 4: Relationship Restructuring

**Evaluating current relationships** helps clients assess which relationships can adapt to include mutual exchange versus those that depend primarily on one-sided caretaking.

**Developing reciprocal relationships** involves learning to both give and receive support rather than maintaining relationships based exclusively on providing care to others.

**Creating authentic connections** means building relationships where you can express your genuine self rather than performing roles designed to maintain others' comfort or approval.

### The Paradox of Authentic Giving

One of the most surprising discoveries for people healing from other-directedness schemas is that learning to include their own needs actually improves their ability to care for others genuinely. The compulsive caretaking driven by schemas often feels burdensome to both the giver and receiver, while chosen generosity feels meaningful and sustainable.

**Sustainable compassion** requires taking care of your own emotional and physical resources so you have genuine energy to offer others. This means saying no to some requests so you can say yes more wholeheartedly to others.

**Authentic helping** comes from choice rather than compulsion. When you help others because you genuinely want to rather than because you fear rejection or conflict, your assistance feels more valuable to both you and them.

**Mutual relationships** become possible when you include your own needs in the equation rather than focusing exclusively on what others want or need. This creates space for others to care for you as well as receive your care.

The healing journey from other-directedness involves discovering that you matter as much as the people you care about. This doesn't mean becoming selfish or inconsiderate—it means including yourself in the circle of people you treat with respect and compassion.

Learning to honor your own voice while maintaining consideration for others represents one of the most challenging but rewarding aspects of trauma recovery. It requires courage to risk disappointing people who have become accustomed to your unlimited availability, but it creates space for relationships based on authentic connection rather than fear-based compliance.

**Fundamental Principles for Reclaiming Your Authentic Self**

- Your needs and feelings matter as much as others' and deserve consideration in relationship decisions

- Saying no to some requests allows you to say yes more genuinely to others

- Conflict doesn't automatically mean rejection and can actually strengthen authentic relationships

- Others are capable of managing their own emotional responses without your constant caretaking

- Sustainable compassion requires including self-care rather than exclusive focus on others

- Authentic relationships include mutual exchange of support rather than one-sided giving

- Learning to disappoint others appropriately creates space for genuine connection based on choice rather than obligation

# Chapter 8: Overvigilance and Inhibition Schemas

The irony of perfectionism hit James with sudden clarity as he sat in his perfectly organized office, surrounded by awards and accolades that felt empty, preparing to deliver his resignation letter. At thirty-five, he had achieved everything he thought he wanted—partner in a prestigious law firm, six-figure income, respect from colleagues and clients. Yet the constant internal pressure to exceed expectations had become unbearable, and the fear of making any mistake had paralyzed his ability to take risks or feel genuine satisfaction from his accomplishments.

James embodied the cruel paradox of overvigilance and inhibition schemas—patterns that often create external success while generating internal misery. These schemas represent the mind's attempt to control unpredictable or dangerous environments through vigilant monitoring and emotional suppression, creating lives that may look admirable from outside while feeling like prisons to those living them.

The four schemas in this domain—negativity/pessimism, emotional inhibition, unrelenting standards, and punitiveness—share a common theme of trying to prevent bad things from happening through constant vigilance and rigid self-control. While these strategies may prevent some problems, they also prevent the spontaneity, emotional connection, and self-compassion necessary for genuine well-being.

## Hypervigilance as a Trauma Response

Hypervigilance represents one of the most common and persistent trauma responses, involving constant scanning of the environment for potential threats or problems. While this response serves essential protective functions in genuinely dangerous situations, it becomes problematic when applied automatically to safe environments or normal life challenges.

**Threat detection systems** in the brain become overactive following trauma, particularly when the trauma involved unpredictable danger or required constant monitoring for safety. The nervous system learns to maintain high alert status, interpreting neutral stimuli as potentially dangerous and normal challenges as catastrophic threats.

Children who grow up in unpredictable environments— homes with addiction, domestic violence, mental illness, or emotional volatility—often develop sophisticated early warning systems that help them navigate family crises. They learn to read subtle cues about adults' emotional states, anticipate problems before they develop, and adjust their behavior to prevent conflicts or disasters.

These skills can be remarkable—trauma survivors often demonstrate exceptional ability to read social dynamics, anticipate others' needs, and respond quickly to changing circumstances. However, the same vigilance that helped them survive childhood can become exhausting and limiting in adult environments that don't require constant threat monitoring.

Consider Rebecca's development of hypervigilance in response to her father's alcoholism and unpredictable rages.

Rebecca learned to monitor his drinking patterns, recognize early signs of anger, and implement damage control strategies that sometimes prevented violent episodes. This hypervigilance helped protect herself and her younger siblings during childhood.

As an adult, Rebecca continued scanning for signs of danger or disapproval in every relationship and work situation. She could predict when her boss was having a bad day, sense tension between friends before they recognized it themselves, and anticipate problems in projects weeks before they materialized. While these skills made her valuable professionally, they also created chronic exhaustion and anxiety that prevented her from enjoying the safety and stability she had worked so hard to create.

Rebecca's hypervigilance manifested as constant worry about potential problems, difficulty relaxing even in safe situations, and physical symptoms like muscle tension and sleep difficulties. She couldn't understand why she felt so anxious when her life was objectively successful and stable—her trauma-adapted nervous system was still operating as if danger lurked around every corner.

**Perfectionism and Emotional Shutdown**

Perfectionism and emotional inhibition often develop together as complementary strategies for maintaining control in chaotic or critical environments. The child who learns that mistakes lead to punishment or rejection may develop both perfectionist standards and emotional suppression as protection against vulnerability.

**Perfectionism** serves multiple functions for trauma survivors. It can prevent criticism, earn approval, create sense of control, and avoid the shame associated with failure or inadequacy. However, perfectionist standards often become so rigid that they prevent risk-taking, creativity, and the trial-and-error learning necessary for growth.

**Emotional inhibition** protects against the vulnerability that comes with authentic emotional expression. Children who learned that emotions were dangerous, burdensome, or used against them may develop sophisticated suppression strategies that persist into adulthood even in emotionally safe relationships.

The combination creates individuals who appear highly competent and controlled while struggling with internal emptiness, relationship difficulties, and inability to experience genuine satisfaction from achievements. They may excel professionally while feeling like frauds, maintain stable relationships while feeling emotionally isolated, and achieve external goals while experiencing little internal joy or fulfillment.

### Case Study: James's Battle with Impossible Standards

James's overvigilance patterns began forming in early childhood through exposure to a family system that valued achievement above emotional well-being and maintained impossibly high standards for performance and behavior.

**Family System Dynamics** James grew up in an upper-middle-class family where both parents worked in demanding professional careers—his father as a surgeon and his mother as a university professor. While his parents provided material security and educational opportunities, they also brought their professional perfectionism into family life.

The family operated more like a high-performing organization than an emotional sanctuary. Dinner conversations focused on achievements and intellectual discussions rather than feelings or personal experiences. James and his sister were expected to excel academically, participate in multiple enrichment activities, and represent the family well in all social situations.

Mistakes or struggles were treated as problems to be solved rather than normal parts of learning and development. When James brought home a B+ grade, the response was analysis of what went wrong rather than celebration of his effort. When he expressed frustration with difficult material, he received tutoring and additional resources rather than comfort and understanding.

**Schema Development** This environment taught James that his worth depended on exceptional performance and that emotions were obstacles to achievement rather than valuable sources of information. He developed unrelenting standards that demanded perfection in every area of life and emotional inhibition that suppressed any feelings that might interfere with performance.

James also developed negativity/pessimism schemas that constantly scanned for potential problems or ways things could go wrong. This vigilance helped him anticipate and prevent many academic and social difficulties, but it also created chronic anxiety and inability to enjoy successes because he was always focused on the next challenge.

**Adult Manifestation** By his thirties, James's schemas had created a life that looked successful from outside while feeling empty and exhausting internally. He worked twelve-hour days not because of external pressure, but because his internal standards demanded excellence that required constant effort. He avoided social situations where he couldn't control outcomes and maintained friendships that felt more like professional networking than genuine connection.

James's romantic relationships suffered because his emotional inhibition prevented the vulnerability necessary for intimacy. He chose partners who appreciated his stability and success but didn't require deep emotional sharing. When relationships did become serious, James's perfectionism created pressure that eventually drove partners away.

**The Breaking Point** James's crisis came when he was offered a promotion to senior partner that would require managing a larger team and taking on more visible leadership responsibilities. Instead of feeling excited about this recognition of his achievements, James experienced panic about the increased opportunities for mistakes and failure.

The realization that success felt as terrifying as failure forced James to confront how his schemas were controlling his life. He recognized that he had built a career around avoiding failure rather than pursuing meaningful goals, and that his emotional inhibition had left him feeling disconnected from both his work and relationships.

**Recovery Process** James's healing journey involved learning to tolerate imperfection while maintaining his natural drive for excellence. This required distinguishing between healthy standards that motivated growth and perfectionist demands that prevented risk-taking and learning.

The process began with small experiments in accepting "good enough" outcomes rather than demanding perfection. James practiced submitting work proposals without endless revisions, participating in social activities where he couldn't control outcomes, and expressing opinions without extensive research and preparation.

Most challenging was developing emotional awareness and expression skills that James had suppressed since childhood. He learned to identify feelings as they arose rather than automatically focusing on tasks and problem-solving. He practiced sharing struggles and uncertainties with trusted friends and eventually with romantic partners.

**Integration and Growth** After two years of conscious work, James reported feeling more engaged with both his work and relationships. He had learned to set challenging but achievable goals rather than impossible standards, and he could experience satisfaction from accomplishments rather than immediately focusing on the next challenge.

Most significantly, James had developed what he called "strategic imperfection"—the ability to choose where to invest his perfectionist energy and where to accept good enough outcomes. This allowed him to maintain his high standards in areas that mattered most while creating space for spontaneity and learning in other areas.

### Learning to Feel Safe with Imperfection

The healing process for overvigilance and inhibition schemas involves developing tolerance for uncertainty, imperfection, and emotional vulnerability while maintaining appropriate caution and standards. This balance requires conscious practice because these schemas often feel essential for safety and success.

**Developing Distress Tolerance**

**Uncertainty tolerance** involves learning to make decisions and take action without guarantees about outcomes. People with overvigilance schemas often delay decisions indefinitely while gathering more information or trying to predict all possible consequences.

Practice making small decisions with incomplete information—choosing restaurants without reading every review, accepting social invitations without knowing everyone who will attend, or starting projects without planning every detail in advance.

**Mistake tolerance** requires developing self-compassion for normal human errors rather than treating every mistake as evidence of inadequacy. This involves learning from errors without excessive self-criticism and recognizing that mistakes are essential for learning and growth.

**Criticism tolerance** means learning to receive feedback without defensive reactions or devastating self-attacks. Practice listening to criticism for useful information while maintaining perspective about your overall competence and worth.

**Emotional Awareness and Expression**

**Feeling identification** forms the foundation of emotional health but can feel threatening to people who learned that emotions were dangerous or disruptive. Start by noticing physical sensations and energy levels throughout the day before trying to identify specific emotions.

**Graduated emotional expression** involves sharing feelings in small doses with safe people rather than continuing to suppress all emotional responses. Begin with positive emotions and minor concerns before attempting to express more vulnerable feelings.

**Emotional acceptance** means learning to experience feelings without immediately trying to change, fix, or justify them. Practice sitting with emotions long enough to understand what they're trying to communicate rather than automatically moving to problem-solving mode.

### Treatment Protocols: Mindfulness and Self-Compassion Approaches

Schema therapy addresses overvigilance and inhibition patterns through approaches that help clients develop present-moment awareness and self-compassion while gradually reducing rigid control strategies.

### Mindfulness-Based Interventions

**Present-moment awareness** helps counteract the hypervigilance tendency to constantly scan for future problems or ruminate about past mistakes. Regular mindfulness practice trains attention to focus on current experience rather than anxious projections or regrets.

**Body awareness** reconnects clients with physical sensations and needs that may have been suppressed through emotional inhibition. This includes noticing tension, fatigue, hunger, and other signals that provide information about emotional and physical well-being.

**Thought observation** involves learning to notice perfectionist and catastrophic thoughts without automatically believing or acting on them. This creates space between thoughts and responses, allowing for more conscious choice about how to interpret and respond to situations.

## Self-Compassion Development

**Self-kindness** involves treating yourself with the same care you would offer a good friend who was struggling. This includes speaking to yourself with kindness during difficulties rather than harsh criticism and self-attack.

**Common humanity** recognition helps you understand that struggles, mistakes, and imperfection are normal parts of human experience rather than evidence of personal inadequacy. This reduces the isolation that often accompanies perfectionist schemas.

**Mindful acceptance** of difficult emotions and experiences allows them to be present without overwhelming you or requiring immediate action. This includes accepting anxiety about imperfection without automatically reverting to perfectionist behaviors.

## Graduated Exposure to Imperfection

**Intentional mistake-making** involves deliberately creating small imperfections to practice tolerating the anxiety that accompanies less-than-perfect outcomes. This might include sending emails with minor typos, submitting work that's good enough rather than perfect, or wearing slightly mismatched clothing.

**Risk-taking practice** helps clients gradually expand their comfort zones by taking on challenges with uncertain outcomes. Start with low-stakes risks like trying new activities or expressing opinions in safe groups before attempting larger risks in career or relationships.

**Spontaneity exercises** counteract the rigid planning and control that characterize overvigilance schemas. Practice making unplanned decisions, accepting last-minute invitations, or changing established routines to build tolerance for unpredictability.

### The Freedom Found in Good Enough

The ultimate goal for healing overvigilance and inhibition schemas isn't to eliminate standards or become careless— it's to develop flexible responses that match the actual demands of each situation rather than applying rigid perfectionism universally.

**Strategic perfectionism** involves choosing where to invest perfectionist energy based on actual importance rather than automatically applying highest standards to every task and situation. This allows you to maintain excellence in areas that truly matter while accepting good enough outcomes elsewhere.

**Emotional intelligence** develops when you can access and use emotional information to make better decisions rather than suppressing feelings that might provide valuable guidance. This includes using anxiety as information about real risks while distinguishing it from schema-driven catastrophic thinking.

**Authentic confidence** emerges when your self-worth isn't dependent on perfect performance or complete control over outcomes. This allows you to take appropriate risks, learn from mistakes, and experience genuine satisfaction from achievements rather than constant focus on what could go wrong.

The journey toward healthy flexibility requires courage because it involves deliberately practicing behaviors that feel dangerous to schemas designed to prevent problems through vigilance and control. However, the freedom that comes from accepting imperfection and embracing emotional authenticity ultimately provides more safety and satisfaction than rigid control strategies ever could.

Learning to feel safe with uncertainty, imperfection, and emotional vulnerability doesn't mean becoming careless or irresponsible. Instead, it means developing wisdom about when vigilance is genuinely needed and when it's schema-driven fear that prevents growth and connection.

Most importantly, healing these patterns opens possibilities for experiencing life with spontaneity, joy, and authentic engagement rather than constant worry about potential problems or mistakes. The energy previously spent on hypervigilance and emotional suppression becomes available for creativity, connection, and genuine satisfaction from life experiences.

**The Path to Balanced Excellence**

Overvigilance and inhibition schemas represent perhaps the most socially rewarded patterns among all early maladaptive schemas. Our culture often celebrates perfectionism, emotional control, and constant vigilance as virtues, making it difficult to recognize when these traits have become problematic.

Yet beneath the external success these patterns can create lies a different reality—chronic anxiety, emotional emptiness, relationship difficulties, and inability to experience genuine satisfaction from achievements. The very strategies that may have helped you survive difficult circumstances and achieve external success can become prisons that prevent authentic living.

Recovery doesn't require abandoning excellence or becoming careless about important responsibilities. Instead, it involves developing the flexibility to match your responses to actual situational demands rather than applying rigid perfectionism and emotional control universally.

The process requires patience because these schemas often feel essential for safety and success. Learning to tolerate imperfection, express emotions authentically, and accept uncertainty can feel terrifying initially. However, the freedom that emerges from this flexibility ultimately provides more genuine safety and satisfaction than rigid control ever could.

As we move forward to explore the dynamic nature of schema modes—the moment-to-moment emotional states that combine schemas with current coping responses— remember that your capacity for vigilance and self-control represents strength that can be redirected rather than eliminated. The same intelligence that created these protective patterns can learn to use them wisely rather than compulsively.

**Core Insights from Overvigilance and Inhibition Patterns**

- Hypervigilance develops as protective response to unpredictable or dangerous environments but becomes limiting in safe situations

- Perfectionism and emotional inhibition often work together to create appearance of success while generating internal suffering

- These patterns are socially rewarded, making them difficult to recognize as problematic

- Recovery involves developing flexibility to match responses to actual situational demands rather than universal rigid control

- Strategic perfectionism allows maintaining excellence in important areas while accepting good enough outcomes elsewhere

- Emotional awareness and expression provide valuable information for decision-making when not suppressed

- Tolerance for uncertainty, imperfection, and vulnerability ultimately provides more safety than rigid control strategies

# Chapter 9: Child Modes in Complex Trauma

The first time Rebecca saw her vulnerable child mode during an imagery exercise, she broke down sobbing in a way that surprised both of us. There, in her mind's eye, was a seven-year-old version of herself—small, frightened, and desperately trying to make sense of why daddy kept hurting mommy and why mommy couldn't protect her. This little girl had been carrying decades of terror, sadness, and confusion while thirty-four-year-old Rebecca went about her successful career as a marketing executive.

"I've been so mean to her," Rebecca whispered through her tears. "I've been telling her to shut up and stop being weak for twenty-seven years." That moment marked the beginning of Rebecca's healing journey—not just understanding her trauma intellectually, but developing a relationship with the wounded parts of herself that had been silenced, criticized, and abandoned in the name of moving forward.

Schema modes represent one of the most powerful aspects of Young's framework because they capture the dynamic, moment-to-moment nature of trauma responses. While schemas operate as stable background patterns, modes shift and change based on triggers, relationships, and circumstances. Child modes—vulnerable child, angry child, impulsive child, and happy child—represent the core emotional experiences that trauma often fragments or suppresses.

## How Trauma Fragments the Child Self

Healthy child development involves integrating different emotional states into a coherent sense of self. Children naturally experience vulnerability, anger, impulsiveness, and joy as part of normal emotional development. They learn to express these feelings appropriately while maintaining connection with caregivers and developing self-regulation skills.

Trauma disrupts this integration process in profound ways. When children experience abuse, neglect, or chronic stress, their emotional states can become **fragmented** rather than integrated. The child learns that some parts of themselves are dangerous, unacceptable, or must be hidden to maintain safety or connection.

Consider how trauma affects each child mode differently. The **vulnerable child** mode—which naturally seeks comfort, protection, and emotional connection—may go underground if expressing vulnerability leads to punishment, rejection, or further harm. The child learns to suppress sadness, fear, and need for comfort because these emotions either don't bring help or actually increase danger.

The **angry child** mode—which naturally responds to injustice, boundary violations, and unmet needs—may become explosive if the child has no safe way to express frustration, or it may become completely suppressed if anger is met with retaliation or abandonment. Some trauma survivors struggle with rage that feels overwhelming and destructive, while others can't access anger even in situations that warrant it.

The **impulsive child** mode—which represents natural spontaneity, playfulness, and immediate emotional expression—often gets severely restricted in traumatic environments. Children may learn that acting on impulses leads to punishment or chaos, creating rigid self-control that continues into adulthood even in safe environments.

Most tragically, the **happy child** mode—representing joy, wonder, creativity, and spontaneous delight—frequently becomes inaccessible following trauma. Children may learn that happiness is dangerous because it makes them vulnerable, that joy is temporary and will inevitably be followed by pain, or that expressing delight brings unwanted attention or jealousy from others.

The fragmentation process creates internal splits where different child modes become isolated from each other and from conscious awareness. An adult trauma survivor might function competently in professional settings while carrying a terrified vulnerable child that never learned safety, an enraged angry child that never experienced justice, and a joyful happy child that learned to hide its light to avoid destruction.

### Accessing the Wounded Inner Child Safely

Working with child modes requires creating safety that many trauma survivors never experienced during childhood. The adult must learn to provide the protection, comfort, and understanding that the child modes desperately need but may have learned to distrust.

**Safety creation** forms the foundation of child mode work. This involves helping the adult part of the person develop capacity to recognize when child modes are activated and respond with compassion rather than criticism or suppression. Many trauma survivors have internalized harsh parental voices that attack vulnerable feelings the same way critical caregivers did.

**Co-regulation skills** help the adult part soothe distressed child modes rather than being overwhelmed by their emotions. This might involve breathing techniques, grounding exercises, or physical comfort measures that help regulate the nervous system when child modes become activated.

**Protective boundaries** ensure that child mode work happens in appropriate contexts rather than exposing vulnerable parts to people or situations that might retraumatize them. The adult learns to distinguish between safe relationships where vulnerability is appropriate and situations where protection is needed.

**Gradual exposure** prevents overwhelming vulnerable child modes with too much attention or emotion too quickly. Some trauma survivors have suppressed child modes so thoroughly that sudden access to these emotions feels terrifying and destabilizing.

Take Jennifer's experience with her vulnerable child mode. After decades of refusing to cry or ask for help, Jennifer's first experience of connecting with her wounded child felt overwhelming and dangerous. She worried that if she started crying, she might never stop. If she acknowledged how much she had needed comfort and protection, she might fall apart completely.

The healing process required Jennifer to practice connecting with her vulnerable child in small doses while maintaining her adult functioning. She might spend ten minutes writing in a journal to her child self, or holding a stuffed animal while listening to music that moved her emotionally, then return to adult activities with conscious intention.

This gradual approach allowed Jennifer's nervous system to learn that accessing child emotions didn't mean losing adult competence or becoming overwhelmed permanently. Over time, she developed capacity to move fluidly between child and adult modes rather than keeping them rigidly separated.

**Case Study: Rebecca's Journey to Healing Her Vulnerable Child**

Rebecca's path to child mode healing illustrates both the challenges and rewards of developing a relationship with wounded inner child parts. Her journey spanned three years and involved multiple phases of recognition, connection, protection, and integration.

**Background and Trauma History** Rebecca grew up in a household where domestic violence was a constant threat. Her father's alcoholism created unpredictable episodes of rage that could be triggered by any perceived disruption to his comfort or authority. Her mother, trapped by financial dependence and her own trauma history, alternated between attempting to protect the children and becoming emotionally unavailable due to depression and fear.

From ages five through fifteen, Rebecca learned to monitor her father's drinking patterns, anticipate his mood changes, and implement damage control strategies that sometimes prevented violent episodes. She became hypervigilant about family emotional dynamics while suppressing her own feelings and needs to avoid creating additional stress.

The vulnerable child part of Rebecca—the part that needed comfort during scary times, reassurance when confused, and protection when threatened—learned that expressing these needs either brought no help or made situations worse. Rebecca's survival strategy involved becoming the family caretaker while banishing her own vulnerability so completely that she lost awareness of it entirely.

**Adult Pattern Recognition** By her thirties, Rebecca had created a successful life that appeared stable and confident. She excelled professionally, maintained active friendships, and presented herself as someone who could handle any challenge independently. Yet she struggled with chronic anxiety, difficulty sleeping, and a sense of emotional emptiness that no external achievement could fill.

Rebecca's relationships suffered because her suppressed vulnerable child created barriers to intimacy. She couldn't ask for comfort during difficult times, express fears or insecurities, or allow others to take care of her emotionally. Partners appreciated her strength and independence but eventually felt shut out by her inability to share struggles or accept support.

The pattern that brought Rebecca to therapy involved panic attacks triggered by her boyfriend's mention of taking a vacation together. The thought of being in an unfamiliar place where she couldn't control the environment activated her vulnerable child's terror, but Rebecca experienced this only as overwhelming anxiety without understanding its source.

**Initial Child Mode Contact** Rebecca's first experience connecting with her vulnerable child happened during a guided imagery exercise where she visualized herself at age seven. The image that emerged was heartbreaking—a small girl sitting alone in her bedroom, listening to her parents fight downstairs, trying not to cry because crying might make daddy angrier.

This little girl was carrying decades of accumulated fear, sadness, and confusion that adult Rebecca had never acknowledged or comforted. The child had been waiting for someone—anyone—to notice her pain and tell her that the fighting wasn't her fault, that she deserved protection, and that her feelings mattered.

Rebecca's initial response was to feel sorry for the child while maintaining emotional distance. "Poor little thing," she said, as if describing someone else's experience. The work involved helping Rebecca recognize that this wasn't a separate person but a part of herself that had been split off and abandoned.

**Developing a Protective Relationship** The next phase involved Rebecca learning to respond to her vulnerable child the way a loving parent would respond to a frightened child. This required developing entirely new internal responses because Rebecca had no template for how to comfort vulnerability—she had only learned to suppress or criticize it.

Rebecca practiced having conversations with her child self, starting with simple acknowledgments: "You were so scared during those fights. It makes sense that you felt terrified. You were just a little kid trying to understand grown-up problems." These conversations felt artificial initially because Rebecca's automatic response was to tell the child to "stop being a baby" or "get over it."

Gradually, Rebecca developed genuine compassion for her child self. She began understanding that her childhood hypervigilance and caretaking represented remarkable intelligence and strength rather than character flaws. The child had developed sophisticated survival strategies that helped protect herself and her family during genuinely dangerous situations.

**Protective Boundary Development** Rebecca learned to distinguish between situations where her vulnerable child could safely emerge and contexts that required adult protection. She practiced accessing vulnerable feelings in therapy, with close friends, and with her boyfriend during calm moments while maintaining adult functioning during work challenges or family conflicts.

This boundary work prevented Rebecca from becoming overwhelmed by child emotions in inappropriate contexts while ensuring that her vulnerable child received the attention and care it needed. Rebecca developed internal signals that helped her recognize when her child mode was activated so she could respond consciously rather than automatically suppressing or being overwhelmed by the emotions.

**Integration and Ongoing Relationship** After two years of conscious child mode work, Rebecca reported feeling more emotionally authentic and connected in her relationships. She could ask for comfort during difficult times, express fears and concerns without shame, and accept care from others without feeling weak or burdensome.

Most significantly, Rebecca's anxiety decreased dramatically as her vulnerable child received the attention and comfort it had been seeking through symptoms. The panic attacks that initially brought her to therapy became rare occurrences rather than regular experiences because Rebecca could recognize and address her child's fears before they escalated to panic levels.

Rebecca described the ongoing relationship with her vulnerable child as "having an internal compass for what I really need." Instead of pushing through all difficulties with rigid independence, she could recognize when she needed support, rest, or comfort and take appropriate action to meet those needs.

**Professional Techniques for Child Mode Work**

Schema therapy has developed specific techniques for safely accessing and healing child modes while maintaining adult functioning and preventing retraumatization. These approaches require specialized training but can be adapted for various clinical contexts.

**Imagery Rescripting for Child Modes**

**Accessing child memories through imagery** allows clients to revisit traumatic experiences while maintaining adult perspective and resources. The technique involves guiding clients into relaxed states where they can visualize themselves as children in problematic situations.

**Rescripting traumatic scenes** involves the adult self entering childhood memories to provide protection, comfort, or justice that wasn't available originally. This might include confronting abusive caregivers, removing the child from dangerous situations, or simply offering comfort and understanding to the frightened child.

**Integration work** helps clients understand how childhood experiences created current patterns while developing new internal responses that support healing rather than perpetuating trauma patterns. The goal isn't to change what happened but to change the child's experience of being alone with trauma.

### Empty Chair Techniques for Child Modes

**Child-adult dialogues** involve clients speaking from both adult and child perspectives to develop internal communication and understanding. The adult learns to listen to the child's feelings and needs while the child learns to trust the adult's protection and wisdom.

**Caregiver confrontation** allows adult clients to express childhood feelings to internal representations of caregivers who caused harm. This technique helps process anger, hurt, and disappointment while maintaining appropriate boundaries with actual family members.

**Protective interventions** involve the adult self setting boundaries with internal critical voices or external people who threaten the child's well-being. Clients practice saying things like "You can't talk to my child that way" or "I won't let anyone hurt this child again."

### Somatic Approaches to Child Mode Healing

**Body awareness** helps clients recognize how child modes show up in physical sensations, posture, and energy levels. Trauma often gets stored in the body, and child modes may carry specific physical patterns that need attention and care.

**Comfort objects** can provide tangible support for child modes during healing work. Some clients benefit from holding stuffed animals, blankets, or other objects that represent safety and care while accessing vulnerable emotions.

**Protective movement** involves using physical positioning to help child modes feel safe and protected. This might include curling up in comfortable positions, creating physical barriers, or practicing protective stances that help the nervous system feel more secure.

### Guided Exercise: Safe Visualization and Inner Child Dialogue

This exercise helps you begin developing a relationship with your child modes in a safe, controlled way. Practice this technique when you're in a calm state and have privacy for emotional processing.

### Preparation Phase

1. **Create physical safety** by choosing a comfortable, private space where you won't be interrupted

2. **Set time boundaries** by deciding how long you'll spend on this exercise (start with 10-15 minutes)

3. **Prepare comfort items** like blankets, pillows, or other objects that help you feel safe

4. **Practice grounding** by noticing five things you can see, four things you can hear, three things you can touch

### Visualization Phase

1. **Close your eyes** and imagine yourself in a safe, peaceful place—this might be a real location or an imaginary sanctuary

2.  **Notice the details** of your safe place—what do you see, hear, smell, or feel?

3.  **Invite your child self** to join you in this safe space— what age does this child appear to be?

4.  **Observe the child** without trying to change anything—what is the child doing, feeling, or needing?

**Dialogue Phase**

1.  **Speak to the child** from your adult self—"Hello, I see you there. I'm here with you now"

2.  **Listen for response**—does the child have anything to say or express?

3.  **Offer comfort** appropriate to what the child needs— this might be words, presence, or imaginary physical comfort

4.  **Ask what the child needs** from you as the adult— protection, understanding, fun, comfort?

5.  **Make a promise** to the child about how you'll treat them going forward

**Integration Phase**

1.  **Thank the child** for trusting you with their feelings and experiences

2.  **Gradually return** to adult awareness while maintaining connection to the child

3.  **Notice any emotions** that arose during the exercise without judging them

4. **Journal briefly** about what you experienced or learned

## Safety Guidelines

- Stop immediately if you feel overwhelmed or disconnected from present reality

- Start with short sessions and gradually increase time as you build tolerance

- Seek professional support if childhood trauma was severe or if this exercise triggers intense reactions

- Practice self-care after child mode work—comfort, rest, or gentle activities

## The Integration of Childlike Wonder and Adult Wisdom

Child mode work isn't about regressing to childish behavior or becoming emotionally immature. Instead, it's about reclaiming authentic emotional experiences that trauma may have suppressed while maintaining adult functioning and judgment. The goal is integration—having access to the full range of human emotions and experiences that make life rich and meaningful.

**Healthy vulnerability** allows you to ask for comfort during difficult times, express fears and concerns appropriately, and accept care from others without feeling weak or burdensome. This doesn't mean becoming dependent or helpless—it means including normal human needs for support and connection in your adult life.

**Appropriate anger** helps you recognize when boundaries are being violated, needs aren't being met, or injustices are occurring. Healthy anger provides energy for problem-solving and self-protection rather than destructive rage or complete suppression of natural assertiveness.

**Spontaneous joy** becomes possible when you can access the happy child mode that delights in simple pleasures, finds wonder in everyday experiences, and expresses enthusiasm without fear of judgment or retaliation. This childlike capacity for joy often gets suppressed by trauma but can be reclaimed through conscious healing work.

**Balanced impulsiveness** allows for spontaneity and creativity while maintaining appropriate judgment about consequences. This means being able to act on positive impulses—trying new experiences, expressing affection, or pursuing interests—without being controlled by destructive impulses or rigid overcontrol.

The journey of healing child modes requires patience because these parts of yourself may have been suppressed or criticized for years or decades. Learning to trust that your emotions matter, that vulnerability can be safe, and that joy is allowable takes time and conscious practice.

Most importantly, child mode healing happens in relationship—both with yourself and with others who can accept and support your authentic emotional expression. The child parts that were wounded in relationship need healing experiences in relationship, whether that's through therapy, friendship, romantic partnership, or other forms of meaningful connection.

**Reconnecting with Your Authentic Self**

The child modes represent the most authentic parts of yourself—the emotions, needs, and experiences that are genuinely yours rather than adaptations to trauma or external expectations. Healing these modes involves reclaiming parts of yourself that may have been hidden so long that you forgot they existed.

This process requires courage because accessing child modes often brings up emotions that have been suppressed for good reasons. The vulnerable child may carry decades of accumulated sadness. The angry child may hold rage about injustices that were never addressed. The happy child may feel cautious about expressing joy that was previously criticized or destroyed.

Yet the freedom that comes from integrating child modes is remarkable. Clients often describe feeling more authentic, emotionally alive, and connected to others once they develop healthy relationships with their child parts. The energy that was previously used to suppress emotions becomes available for creativity, connection, and genuine engagement with life.

The work continues throughout life because different situations may activate different child modes, and new life experiences may require renegotiating the relationship between adult and child parts. But once you learn to recognize and respond to your child modes with compassion rather than criticism, you have tools for maintaining emotional authenticity regardless of what challenges arise.

**Essential Lessons from Child Mode Healing**

- Trauma fragments natural child emotions that need integration rather than elimination

- Each child mode—vulnerable, angry, impulsive, and happy—serves important functions for emotional health

- Healing requires developing internal safety and protection that may not have existed during childhood

- Child mode work happens gradually to prevent overwhelming suppressed emotions

- Integration allows access to full emotional range while maintaining adult functioning

- The goal is emotional authenticity and aliveness rather than childish regression

- Healing child modes provides foundation for genuine intimacy and life satisfaction

# Chapter 10: Dysfunctional Coping Modes

Alex sat across from me describing his life with the emotional tone of someone reading a grocery list. His voice remained steady as he explained how his marriage was falling apart, his teenage daughter barely spoke to him, and his successful consulting business felt meaningless. "I don't feel sad about any of it," he said matter-of-factly. "I don't really feel anything at all. It's like I'm watching someone else's life through glass."

What Alex described perfectly captured the detached protector mode—one of three dysfunctional coping modes that trauma survivors develop to manage overwhelming emotions and threatening situations. These modes—compliant surrenderer, detached protector, and overcompensator—represent sophisticated survival strategies that helped people navigate dangerous or chaotic environments but become problematic when applied to safe adult relationships and situations.

Unlike child modes, which represent authentic emotional experiences, coping modes are strategic responses designed to minimize pain, avoid conflict, or maintain some sense of control in difficult circumstances. They worked well enough to ensure survival, but they often prevent the authentic connection and emotional engagement necessary for thriving in adult life.

## Survival Strategies That Become Problems

Coping modes develop as intelligent adaptations to environments where authentic emotional expression feels dangerous or futile. Children who experience trauma often discover that certain responses help them navigate family crises, avoid punishment, or maintain some connection with caregivers who are struggling with their own problems.

**The compliant surrenderer mode** emerges when children learn that survival depends on avoiding conflict at all costs. These children become experts at reading others' moods, anticipating needs, and adjusting their behavior to maintain harmony. While this strategy may prevent abuse or abandonment, it also requires suppressing authentic feelings and preferences completely.

Consider Sarah's development of compliant surrenderer mode in response to her mother's severe mental illness. Sarah learned that any expression of needs, opinions, or emotions could trigger her mother's psychotic episodes or suicidal threats. To maintain some sense of safety and connection, Sarah became a perfectly agreeable child who never disagreed, complained, or asked for anything.

This strategy helped Sarah survive a chaotic childhood, but it created lasting patterns that interfered with adult relationships. Sarah continued suppressing her authentic self even in safe relationships, automatically agreeing with others' preferences while losing touch with her own feelings and desires.

**The detached protector mode** develops when children learn that emotional connection leads to pain, disappointment, or vulnerability that feels unbearable. These children protect themselves by numbing emotions, maintaining distance from others, and focusing on activities that don't require emotional risk.

Alex's detached protector mode formed during years of watching his alcoholic father's emotional volatility terrorize the family. Alex learned that caring deeply about anything—relationships, hopes, achievements—only led to disappointment when his father's drinking destroyed family plans, special occasions, and moments of connection.

To protect himself from ongoing disappointment and pain, Alex developed the ability to disconnect emotionally from people and situations that mattered to him. This emotional numbing helped him function during childhood chaos, but it also prevented him from experiencing joy, intimacy, or genuine satisfaction from relationships and achievements.

**The overcompensator mode** emerges when children learn that they can earn safety, love, or respect by being exceptional in some way. These children may become high achievers, caretakers, entertainers, or rebels—whatever role seems to provide some power or protection in their particular family system.

Jennifer's overcompensator mode developed as a response to emotional neglect and criticism from parents who seemed to notice her only when she excelled academically or helped manage family responsibilities. Jennifer learned that ordinary efforts or normal childhood needs brought indifference or criticism, while exceptional performance earned temporary approval and attention.

This strategy helped Jennifer succeed academically and professionally, but it also created exhausting patterns of perfectionism and workaholism that prevented her from experiencing relationships or activities that didn't involve achievement or caretaking.

## Understanding Dissociation and Emotional Numbing

Dissociation represents one of the most common coping strategies trauma survivors develop, particularly those who experienced chronic or severe abuse during childhood. This natural protective mechanism allows people to mentally disconnect from overwhelming experiences, but it can become automatic and interfere with normal life functioning.

**Mild dissociation** might involve spacing out during stressful conversations, feeling detached from your body during medical procedures, or experiencing emotional numbness during conflict. These responses can be protective in genuinely threatening situations but become problematic when they occur automatically in safe contexts.

**Moderate dissociation** can include feeling like you're watching yourself from outside your body, experiencing gaps in memory during stressful events, or feeling like other people and situations aren't quite real. These experiences often develop during childhood trauma and continue as automatic responses to stress or emotional intensity.

**Severe dissociation** may involve complete disconnection from memory, identity, or physical sensations during traumatic experiences. While this level of dissociation can be essential for psychological survival during severe trauma, it often requires professional treatment to prevent interference with daily functioning.

Understanding dissociation helps explain why some trauma survivors describe feeling "empty," "numb," or "like robots" even when their lives appear successful and stable. The protective numbing that helped them survive trauma continues operating even in safe circumstances, preventing access to the full range of emotions necessary for life satisfaction.

The challenge involves learning to recognize when dissociation is happening and developing skills for returning to present-moment awareness and emotional connection. This process requires patience because the nervous system learned to disconnect for protective reasons and may initially resist efforts to reconnect.

### Case Study: Alex's Pattern of Emotional Detachment

Alex's journey from emotional disconnection to authentic engagement illustrates both the protective function of detached protector mode and the gradual process required for learning to reconnect with feelings and relationships.

**Childhood Development of Detachment** Alex grew up as the oldest of three children in a family dominated by his father's alcoholism and his mother's chronic depression. His father's drinking created unpredictable cycles of rage, remorse, and emotional unavailability that made normal family life impossible. His mother, overwhelmed by her husband's addiction and her own mental health struggles, alternated between emotional clinging and complete withdrawal.

From ages eight through eighteen, Alex learned that emotional investment in family relationships led to constant disappointment and pain. Special occasions got ruined by his father's drinking. Promises were broken regularly. Moments of connection were followed by emotional abandonment when his parents retreated into their own problems.

Alex's survival strategy involved developing the ability to disconnect emotionally from situations and people that mattered to him. He could participate in family activities without expecting them to go well. He could care about his parents without being devastated by their inability to provide consistent love and support. He could pursue goals and relationships without investing enough emotion to be truly hurt by failures or rejections.

This emotional detachment helped Alex function as the responsible older brother who managed practical tasks and looked after younger siblings when his parents couldn't. It also helped him excel academically because he could work hard without being emotionally invested in outcomes that might be influenced by family chaos.

**Adult Pattern Manifestation** By his forties, Alex had created what appeared to be a successful life—a thriving business, a twenty-year marriage, two children, and a reputation as someone who could handle any crisis calmly and effectively. Yet underneath this apparent success, Alex felt emotionally empty and disconnected from the life he had built.

Alex's marriage suffered because his emotional detachment prevented genuine intimacy. His wife appreciated his stability and reliability but felt lonely in the relationship because Alex never shared struggles, fears, or dreams. He participated in family activities efficiently but without apparent joy or enthusiasm.

His children experienced him as a competent provider who was emotionally unavailable for deeper connection. Alex attended their school events and managed practical needs but couldn't engage with their emotional experiences or share in their excitement about achievements and interests.

Professionally, Alex's detachment served him well in crisis management but prevented him from experiencing satisfaction from successes or learning from failures. He completed projects competently but felt no sense of accomplishment or engagement with his work.

**Recognition and Crisis** Alex's crisis began when his wife threatened divorce and his teenage daughter told him she felt like she didn't have a real father. These confrontations forced Alex to recognize that his protective emotional detachment was preventing him from having the relationships and life experiences he actually wanted.

The turning point came when Alex realized he couldn't remember the last time he had felt genuine excitement, joy, sadness, or anger about anything important in his life. His protective numbing had become so automatic that he had lost access to most emotions, not just the painful ones he originally wanted to avoid.

**Therapeutic Process** Alex's healing journey involved learning to reconnect with emotions gradually while developing tolerance for the vulnerability that comes with emotional engagement. This process required patience because his nervous system had learned to disconnect automatically whenever emotional intensity arose.

The work began with helping Alex recognize when his detached protector mode was activated versus when he was genuinely present and engaged. Alex learned to notice physical sensations, energy levels, and emotional responses that he had been suppressing for decades.

Gradually, Alex practiced staying emotionally present during low-risk situations—conversations with friends, enjoyable activities, moments of physical pleasure or comfort. He learned grounding techniques that helped him remain connected to his body and emotions rather than automatically spacing out when feelings arose.

**Relationship Reconnection** The most challenging aspect of Alex's healing involved learning to be emotionally present with his family members who had adapted to his emotional unavailability. His wife initially felt skeptical about his attempts to engage more emotionally because she had protected herself from disappointment by expecting nothing from him emotionally.

Alex had to practice expressing feelings, asking about others' emotional experiences, and sharing his internal responses to family events and conversations. These interactions felt artificial initially because Alex had no template for emotional engagement—he had to learn skills that most people develop during childhood.

Over time, Alex's family began responding to his increased emotional availability. His relationship with his wife deepened as they began sharing struggles and dreams rather than just managing practical responsibilities. His relationship with his children improved as he became curious about their emotional experiences and began sharing his own feelings about their achievements and challenges.

**Professional and Life Integration** After three years of conscious work on emotional reconnection, Alex reported feeling more engaged with all aspects of his life. He could experience genuine satisfaction from business successes and learn from failures without being overwhelmed. He chose projects based on interest and meaning rather than just efficiency and competence.

Most significantly, Alex regained access to the full spectrum of human emotions—joy, sadness, anger, fear, excitement, and love. While this sometimes felt overwhelming, Alex appreciated feeling truly alive and engaged with his life rather than watching it from emotional distance.

### Professional Interventions for Coping Mode Modification

Schema therapy approaches dysfunctional coping modes through interventions designed to help clients recognize when these modes are activated and develop alternative responses that serve current life circumstances rather than childhood survival needs.

### Assessment and Recognition Techniques

**Mode monitoring** helps clients identify when they shift into coping modes versus when they're operating from authentic emotional states. This involves tracking patterns around different triggers, relationships, and life situations that activate protective responses.

**Somatic awareness** training helps clients recognize how different modes feel in their bodies. Compliant surrenderer might feel like physical shrinking or chest tightness. Detached protector often involves numbing, disconnection, or feeling "spacey." Overcompensator might create physical tension, urgency, or driven energy.

**Trigger identification** involves mapping the specific situations, relationships, and emotional states that automatically activate coping modes. Understanding these patterns helps clients develop conscious choice about when protective responses are genuinely needed versus when they're schema-driven habits.

**Cognitive Interventions for Mode Flexibility**

**Cost-benefit analysis** helps clients examine how coping modes served them historically versus how they affect current life circumstances. This balanced approach acknowledges the intelligence of these strategies while recognizing their current limitations.

**Reality testing** involves examining whether current situations actually require the protective responses that worked during childhood. Clients learn to distinguish between genuine threats that warrant protection and safe circumstances where authentic engagement is possible.

**Alternative response development** helps clients create new choices for handling triggering situations. Instead of automatically entering coping modes, clients develop repertoires of responses that match actual circumstances rather than childhood survival needs.

**Experiential and Behavioral Interventions**

**Graduated exposure** to emotional engagement helps clients practice staying present and authentic in low-risk situations before attempting emotional availability in more challenging relationships or circumstances.

**Mindfulness practices** help clients develop present-moment awareness that counteracts the disconnection and numbness characteristic of many coping modes. Regular mindfulness practice strengthens capacity for staying grounded during emotional intensity.

**Relationship experiments** involve practicing authentic engagement in safe relationships while maintaining appropriate boundaries. Clients learn to express genuine feelings, needs, and preferences rather than automatically suppressing them to maintain harmony or safety.

## Self-Assessment: Identifying Your Dominant Coping Modes

Understanding your personal coping mode patterns provides foundation for developing more flexible responses to challenging situations. Complete this assessment honestly, recognizing that most people use multiple coping modes depending on circumstances.

### Compliant Surrenderer Mode Assessment

Rate how often these patterns apply to you (never, sometimes, often, almost always):

- I automatically agree with others even when I have different opinions

- I suppress my needs and preferences to avoid conflict

- I feel responsible for managing others' emotions and comfort

- I have difficulty saying no to requests even when I'm overwhelmed

- I often don't know what I want because I focus on what others want

- I feel anxious or guilty when others seem upset or disappointed

- I change my behavior based on others' moods and reactions

- I rarely express anger or disagreement directly

## Detached Protector Mode Assessment

Rate how often these patterns apply to you:

- I feel emotionally numb or disconnected from my feelings

- I space out or disconnect during stressful or emotional situations

- I avoid activities or relationships that might lead to disappointment

- I feel like I'm watching my life from outside rather than fully living it

- I have difficulty experiencing joy, excitement, or enthusiasm

- I maintain emotional distance even in close relationships

- I focus on practical tasks rather than emotional experiences

- I feel empty or bored even when my life is going well

## Overcompensator Mode Assessment

Rate how often these patterns apply to you:

- I work excessively hard to prove my worth and competence

- I take on leadership roles and responsibilities automatically

- I feel driven to achieve or excel in most areas of my life

- I become impatient with others who don't meet my standards

- I have difficulty relaxing or doing activities that aren't productive

- I feel like I need to be the best or most capable person in most situations

- I take charge of situations even when others could handle them

- I feel restless or anxious when I'm not accomplishing something

**Integration and Interpretation**

Most people show patterns from multiple coping modes, and the same person might use different modes in different circumstances. The goal isn't to eliminate these responses entirely but to develop conscious choice about when they're genuinely helpful versus when they're automatic habits that limit your life.

**High scores in compliant surrenderer** suggest you may have learned that peace and safety depend on suppressing your authentic self to maintain others' comfort. Healing involves developing capacity to express your needs and opinions while maintaining consideration for others.

**High scores in detached protector** indicate you may have learned that emotional engagement leads to pain or disappointment. Recovery involves gradually reconnecting with feelings while developing tolerance for the vulnerability that comes with caring about people and outcomes.

**High scores in overcompensator** suggest you may have learned that worth and safety depend on exceptional performance or control. Healing involves developing self-worth that isn't dependent on achievement while maintaining healthy ambition and responsibility.

### The Journey from Survival to Authenticity

Dysfunctional coping modes represent some of humanity's most creative survival strategies—sophisticated ways of navigating impossible circumstances while maintaining some sense of safety and identity. These modes deserve respect for the protection they provided during times when authentic emotional expression might have been genuinely dangerous.

The challenge lies in learning when these protective responses serve current circumstances versus when they prevent the emotional engagement and authentic connection necessary for life satisfaction. This discrimination requires developing present-moment awareness that can assess actual safety rather than automatically assuming danger based on childhood learning.

**Flexibility** becomes the goal rather than elimination of protective responses. Sometimes detachment protects you during genuinely overwhelming situations. Sometimes compliance prevents unnecessary conflict. Sometimes overcompensation helps you handle crises effectively. The key is conscious choice rather than automatic activation.

**Integration** involves maintaining access to protective strategies while developing capacity for authentic emotional engagement when circumstances support it. This means being able to disconnect when necessary while staying present when safe, accommodating others when appropriate while expressing your own needs, and working hard when needed while relaxing when possible.

The journey from coping modes to authentic living requires patience because these patterns often developed over years or decades and feel essential for safety. Learning to trust that authentic emotional expression can be safe, that relationships can handle your genuine feelings, and that you can manage difficult emotions without automatically protecting yourself takes time and supportive relationships.

Most importantly, healing dysfunctional coping modes happens in relationship with others who can accept and support your authentic emotional expression. The same nervous system that learned to protect itself through disconnection, compliance, or overcompensation can learn new patterns through experiencing safety, acceptance, and genuine connection with others.

**Building Bridges to Authentic Living**

The process of healing dysfunctional coping modes involves building bridges between the protective strategies that helped you survive and the authentic engagement that allows you to thrive. This isn't about abandoning protection entirely but about developing the wisdom to know when protection is genuinely needed versus when it's an automatic habit that prevents genuine living.

The most profound shift happens when you realize that the very qualities that make coping modes problematic in safe relationships—emotional distance, automatic compliance, relentless achievement—also represent remarkable adaptability and intelligence. The person who learned to detach during family chaos developed sophisticated emotion regulation skills. The person who became compliant to avoid conflict learned exceptional social sensitivity. The person who overcompensated through achievement developed remarkable persistence and competence.

Recovery involves redirecting these strengths rather than eliminating them. Emotional regulation skills become tools for staying present during challenging conversations rather than disconnecting entirely. Social sensitivity becomes the foundation for genuine empathy rather than automatic self-suppression. Achievement orientation becomes selective excellence rather than compulsive perfectionism.

The goal isn't to become a different person but to become more fully yourself—someone who can access both protective strategies when genuinely needed and authentic emotional engagement when circumstances support it. This integration creates a richness and flexibility that serves both your need for safety and your desire for meaningful connection and life satisfaction.

**Core Principles for Transforming Coping Patterns**

- Coping modes developed as intelligent adaptations that deserve respect rather than criticism

- Recognition of mode activation provides the foundation for developing conscious choice

- Current safety assessment helps distinguish between appropriate protection and automatic habits

- Gradual practice in low-risk situations builds tolerance for authentic emotional engagement

- The goal is flexibility and choice rather than elimination of all protective responses

- Integration honors both your need for safety and your desire for authentic living

- Healing happens through experiencing relationships that can handle your genuine emotional expression

# Chapter 11: Dysfunctional Parent Modes

The voice in Lisa's head was so familiar she barely noticed it anymore—a constant stream of criticism that followed her throughout each day like a cruel companion she couldn't escape. "You're going to be late again because you can't manage your time properly." "Everyone at the meeting could tell you had no idea what you were talking about." "You call that dinner? No wonder your family doesn't appreciate you." The voice sounded exactly like her mother's sharp tone, but it had become so internalized that Lisa experienced it as her own thoughts rather than recognizing it as an unwelcome intrusion.

When Lisa first learned about dysfunctional parent modes in therapy, she felt a mixture of relief and horror. Relief because she finally understood that the harsh internal voice wasn't her authentic self-assessment but a trauma response. Horror because she realized she had been treating herself with the same cruelty her mother had shown her for over thirty years—long after she had moved away from home and built an independent life.

Dysfunctional parent modes—the punitive parent and demanding parent—represent one of schema therapy's most powerful insights: trauma survivors often internalize the voices and messages of caregivers who were critical, demanding, abusive, or emotionally unavailable. These internalized voices continue operating in adulthood, creating ongoing self-attack and impossible standards that prevent healing and authentic self-expression.

**Internalizing Abusive or Demanding Caregivers**

Children naturally internalize aspects of their caregivers as part of normal development. In healthy families, children develop internal voices that provide comfort during stress, guidance during challenges, and encouragement during struggles. These internalized "good enough" parents help children regulate emotions, make decisions, and maintain self-worth when external support isn't available.

Trauma disrupts this internalization process in profound ways. Children who experience criticism, emotional abuse, neglect, or impossible standards often internalize these negative experiences as internal voice patterns that continue the original harm long after the child has grown up and left the traumatic environment.

**The punitive parent mode** develops when children experience harsh criticism, punishment, blame, or emotional abuse from caregivers. This internalized voice continues attacking the person's self-worth, decisions, and efforts with the same cruelty the original caregiver displayed. The punitive parent creates shame, self-attack, and perfectionist demands that can never be satisfied.

Consider how Michael internalized his father's harsh criticism and explosive anger. Michael's father, who struggled with his own unresolved trauma and alcohol abuse, consistently responded to Michael's normal childhood mistakes with rage, criticism, and messages about his inadequacy. "You can't do anything right!" "What's wrong with you?" "You're just like your lazy uncle—you'll never amount to anything!"

These messages became so deeply internalized that Michael continued hearing them in his own voice decades later. When he made mistakes at work, forgot appointments, or struggled with challenges, the punitive parent voice would attack with the same viciousness his father had shown. This internal voice prevented Michael from learning from mistakes, taking appropriate risks, or developing self-compassion.

**The demanding parent mode** emerges when children grow up with caregivers who communicate impossible standards, conditional love, or constant pressure to achieve or behave perfectly. This internalized voice creates relentless pressure to excel, work harder, do more, and meet standards that can never quite be reached.

Sarah's demanding parent mode developed from well-intentioned but impossible messages from parents who wanted her to succeed. Her parents, both professionals who had worked extremely hard to create financial security, consistently communicated that good wasn't good enough, that she should always strive for more, and that rest or satisfaction were signs of complacency.

These messages created an internal voice that drove Sarah to work sixty-hour weeks, exercise obsessively, maintain a perfect home, and achieve in multiple areas simultaneously. The demanding parent never allowed satisfaction or rest because there was always more that could be accomplished, improved, or achieved.

### The Critical Inner Voice in Trauma Survivors

The critical inner voice represents one of the most painful and persistent aspects of trauma recovery because it operates constantly and feels like your own authentic assessment rather than an internalized trauma response. This voice often feels more real and believable than external criticism because it knows your most intimate fears, failures, and vulnerabilities.

**Shame-based messaging** forms the core of punitive parent functioning. This voice doesn't just criticize specific behaviors or mistakes—it attacks your fundamental worth as a person. "You're stupid," "You're disgusting," "You're a failure," "Nobody could love someone like you." These messages create deep shame that affects every aspect of self-perception and life choices.

**Perfectionist demands** characterize the demanding parent voice. This voice sets standards that are impossible to meet and then criticizes you for falling short. "You should have done better," "Everyone else is more successful than you," "If you really cared, you would work harder," "You're being lazy and selfish."

**Comparative criticism** involves the internal voice constantly measuring your efforts, achievements, and worth against others. This voice finds evidence of your inadequacy in others' successes and never allows you to appreciate your own accomplishments because someone else has always done better.

**Future catastrophizing** involves the critical voice predicting terrible outcomes based on current mistakes or struggles. "You're going to fail and everyone will know you're incompetent," "You'll end up alone because you're too damaged for anyone to love," "You'll never amount to anything because you can't even handle simple tasks."

The persistence and intensity of these internal voices often surprises trauma survivors who thought that leaving abusive environments would end the harm. Learning that the abuse has become internalized and continues operating independently can feel overwhelming and discouraging initially.

However, understanding the critical voice as a trauma response rather than authentic self-assessment opens possibilities for healing that wouldn't exist if these patterns were viewed as accurate self-perception. The same neuroplasticity that allowed internalization of critical voices can support developing internal voices that are compassionate, realistic, and supportive.

### Case Study: Lisa's Struggle with Her Internalized Critic

Lisa's journey from self-attack to self-compassion illustrates both the pervasive nature of internalized critical voices and the systematic work required to develop healthier internal dialogue patterns.

**Development of the Critical Voice** Lisa grew up with a mother who struggled with severe anxiety and depression following her own childhood trauma. Lisa's mother had never learned healthy coping strategies or received treatment for her mental health conditions, creating a household environment where emotional volatility and criticism were constant features of daily life.

Lisa's mother's criticism took multiple forms. Sometimes it was explosive—screaming about Lisa's messiness, carelessness, or failure to anticipate her mother's needs. Other times it was subtle but persistent—sighing about Lisa's choices, making comparisons to other children who were "more considerate" or "more responsible," or expressing disappointment about Lisa's achievements.

Most damaging was her mother's tendency to attack Lisa's character rather than addressing specific behaviors. Instead of saying "Please clean up your room," Lisa's mother would say "You're such a slob, just like your father." Instead of helping with homework struggles, she would say "You're not applying yourself—you could do better if you really tried."

These messages taught Lisa that she was fundamentally flawed, that her efforts were never sufficient, and that love and approval depended on meeting impossible standards of behavior and achievement. The criticism became so constant that Lisa internalized the voice and began attacking herself even when her mother wasn't present.

**Adult Manifestation** By her thirties, Lisa had achieved significant external success—a master's degree, a responsible job in healthcare, a stable marriage, and two children. Yet she felt constantly inadequate and overwhelmed because her internalized critical voice made every achievement feel insufficient and every mistake feel catastrophic.

Lisa's self-attack was relentless and pervasive. She criticized her parenting decisions, her professional performance, her appearance, her housekeeping, her relationships, and her emotional responses to stress. The voice was particularly harsh when Lisa was tired, stressed, or facing new challenges.

The critical voice prevented Lisa from enjoying her accomplishments or learning from mistakes in healthy ways. When she received positive feedback at work, the voice dismissed it as politeness or suggested that she had fooled people temporarily. When she made mistakes, the voice attacked her character rather than focusing on problem-solving or learning.

Most painfully, Lisa found herself using the same critical tone with her children that her mother had used with her. Despite her conscious intention to be a supportive parent, Lisa heard herself making sarcastic comments, expressing disappointment about normal childhood behaviors, and setting impossible standards for her children's performance and behavior.

**Recognition and Separation** Lisa's healing began when her therapist helped her recognize the critical voice as an internalized trauma response rather than accurate self-assessment. This involved learning to distinguish between the harsh, attacking tone of her mother's voice and her own authentic thoughts and feelings about situations.

Initially, this distinction felt artificial because the critical voice had operated so long that Lisa experienced it as her natural response to stress and challenges. She had to practice asking herself: "Is this how I would talk to a friend who was facing this same situation?" and "Does this voice sound encouraging and helpful or attacking and shaming?"

Lisa learned to recognize the specific phrases, tone, and content that characterized her mother's critical voice versus her own authentic responses. The critical voice used absolute language ("always," "never," "completely"), attacked her character rather than addressing specific behaviors, and predicted catastrophic outcomes based on minor mistakes.

**Developing Alternative Internal Voices** The next phase involved Lisa practicing alternative internal responses that were realistic but compassionate. Instead of "You're such an idiot for forgetting that appointment," Lisa learned to say, "You made a mistake because you're managing a lot right now. How can you handle this situation and prevent it in the future?"

This process felt uncomfortable initially because Lisa had learned to equate self-criticism with motivation and self-awareness. She worried that being kind to herself would make her lazy, careless, or self-indulgent. Learning that self-compassion actually supports better decision-making and problem-solving required both intellectual understanding and practical experience.

Lisa practiced developing what she called her "wise adult voice"—an internal presence that could assess situations realistically, acknowledge both strengths and areas for growth, and provide guidance without attack or shame. This voice sounded more like a supportive mentor than a harsh critic.

**Integration and Boundary Setting** After two years of conscious work, Lisa reported a dramatic reduction in the frequency and intensity of self-attack. She had learned to recognize critical voice activation and could often shift to more compassionate internal dialogue before the attack escalated.

Most significantly, Lisa had begun setting boundaries with the critical voice rather than automatically believing its assessments. She developed phrases like "That's not helpful right now" or "I'm not going to talk to myself that way" that helped interrupt self-attack patterns before they gained momentum.

Lisa also noticed improvements in her parenting as she became less critical of herself. She could respond to her children's mistakes with patience and problem-solving rather than criticism and disappointment. Breaking the cycle of critical voice transmission became one of her strongest motivations for continuing the healing work.

**Professional Techniques for Parent Mode Work**

Schema therapy has developed specific interventions for addressing dysfunctional parent modes, recognizing that these internalized voices often require different approaches than other trauma responses because they operate continuously and feel like authentic self-assessment.

**Voice Recognition and Separation Techniques**

**Voice mapping** involves helping clients identify the specific content, tone, and phrases that characterize their critical internal voices versus their authentic thoughts and feelings. This often involves tracing the origins of specific phrases or attitudes back to original caregivers.

**Dialogue techniques** help clients practice having conversations between their critical voice and their authentic adult self. This externalization makes it easier to recognize the critical voice as a trauma response rather than accurate self-assessment.

**Historical analysis** involves exploring how critical messages served functions in the original family environment— perhaps protecting the child from worse abuse or helping them maintain some connection with critical caregivers. Understanding these original functions reduces shame about having internalized critical voices.

### Cognitive Restructuring for Critical Voices

**Reality testing** helps clients examine whether their critical voice assessments are accurate, helpful, or proportionate to actual situations. Most critical voices use exaggerated language and predict catastrophic outcomes that don't match reality.

**Alternative perspective development** involves creating internal voices that can assess situations realistically without attack or shame. Clients practice internal dialogue that acknowledges mistakes or areas for growth while maintaining basic respect and compassion.

**Compassionate reframing** helps clients learn to respond to mistakes, challenges, and failures the way they would respond to a good friend facing similar difficulties. This provides a template for internal dialogue that is both honest and supportive.

### Experiential Interventions for Parent Mode Healing

**Empty chair work** allows clients to externalize critical voices and practice setting boundaries or expressing anger about the harm these voices have caused. This technique helps clients distinguish between themselves and the internalized critical voices.

**Imagery rescripting** can involve visualizing conversations with original critical caregivers where the adult self sets boundaries, expresses anger about harmful treatment, or provides protection for their child self. This work helps separate current self-worth from childhood messages.

**Self-compassion practices** help clients develop alternative internal voices that provide comfort, encouragement, and realistic guidance during challenging situations. These practices require repetition because critical voices often resist being replaced by more compassionate alternatives.

## Cognitive Exercise: Challenging the Inner Critic

This structured exercise helps you develop skills for recognizing and responding to critical internal voices in more helpful ways. Practice this technique daily to build new internal dialogue patterns.

### Step 1: Critical Voice Recognition

When you notice self-critical thoughts arising, pause and examine the content:

**Voice characteristics to notice:**

- Absolute language (always, never, completely, totally)

- Character attacks (you're stupid, you're worthless, you're a failure)

- Catastrophic predictions (you'll never succeed, everyone will reject you)

- Comparisons to others (everyone else is better than you)

- Impossible standards (you should be perfect, you should never struggle)

**Origin identification:**

- Does this voice sound like a specific person from your past?

- What phrases or tone remind you of critical caregivers?

- When did you first learn to talk to yourself this way?

**Step 2: Reality Testing**

Challenge the critical voice with specific questions:

**Accuracy assessment:**

- Is this criticism based on facts or feelings?
- Would a neutral observer agree with this assessment?
- Am I using extreme language that doesn't match reality?

**Helpfulness evaluation:**

- Is this internal dialogue helping me solve problems or just creating shame?
- Would I talk to a friend this way if they faced this same situation?
- What would be a more helpful way to address this challenge?

**Proportionality check:**

- Is my emotional response proportionate to what actually happened?
- Am I treating a small mistake like a major catastrophe?
- What would be a realistic consequence for this situation?

**Step 3: Compassionate Alternative Development**

Create internal dialogue that is honest but supportive:

**Acknowledge reality without attack:**

- "I made a mistake because I'm human and humans make mistakes"
- "This is challenging for me right now, and that's understandable"
- "I'm learning and growing, which involves some struggles along the way"

**Focus on problem-solving:**

- "What can I learn from this situation?"
- "How can I handle this differently next time?"
- "What support or resources might help me with this challenge?"

**Maintain perspective:**

- "This is one situation, not a reflection of my entire worth as a person"
- "I've handled difficult things before and can handle this too"
- "My mistakes don't define me—my efforts to learn and grow do"

**Step 4: Daily Practice Integration**

**Morning intention setting:** Begin each day by committing to notice and challenge critical voice activation when it occurs.

**Midday check-ins:** Pause periodically to assess your internal dialogue and redirect criticism toward compassion when needed.

**Evening reflection:** Review moments when you successfully challenged critical voices and moments when you got caught in self-attack patterns.

**Weekly progress assessment:** Notice changes in the frequency, intensity, and believability of critical internal voices over time.

### The Liberation from Internal Tyranny

Healing dysfunctional parent modes represents one of the most liberating aspects of trauma recovery because it addresses the source of ongoing self-harm that can persist long after external threats have ended. Learning to recognize critical voices as trauma responses rather than authentic self-assessment creates possibilities for developing internal relationships based on compassion rather than attack.

The process requires patience because critical voices often resist being replaced by more compassionate alternatives. These voices may have operated for decades and feel essential for motivation, protection, or maintaining connection with original caregivers. Learning to function with self-compassion rather than self-attack can feel foreign and dangerous initially.

Yet the freedom that comes from developing supportive internal dialogue is remarkable. Clients often describe feeling like they've been released from prison when they learn to treat themselves with basic kindness and respect. The energy that was previously used for self-attack becomes available for problem-solving, creativity, and authentic engagement with life challenges.

Most importantly, healing critical internal voices prevents transmission of these patterns to others—children, partners, friends, and colleagues who might otherwise become targets of the same criticism that trauma survivors learned to direct toward themselves. Breaking cycles of criticism and shame represents one of the most powerful gifts trauma survivors can give to their communities and future generations.

The journey toward internal compassion doesn't require eliminating all self-assessment or becoming unrealistic about challenges and areas for growth. Instead, it involves learning to evaluate yourself and your efforts with the same basic respect and kindness you would offer to any other human being facing similar circumstances.

**Building Blocks for Internal Compassion**

- Critical voices represent internalized trauma responses rather than accurate self-assessment

- Recognition and separation from critical voices provides foundation for developing healthier internal dialogue

- Self-compassion supports better decision-making and problem-solving than self-attack

- Challenging critical voices requires daily practice and conscious attention to internal dialogue patterns

- The goal is realistic self-assessment combined with basic kindness and respect

- Healing critical voices prevents transmission of these patterns to others in your life

- Internal compassion provides foundation for authentic relationships and life satisfaction

# Chapter 12: The Healthy Adult Mode

Michael's transformation didn't happen overnight, but the moment he recognized it was unmistakable. He was sitting in a difficult meeting where a colleague was criticizing a project he had managed, and instead of his usual responses—either defending aggressively or shutting down completely—he found himself listening carefully, asking clarifying questions, and acknowledging the valid points while maintaining confidence in his overall competence. "I can see why you're concerned about the timeline," he said calmly. "Let me think about how we can address those issues while keeping the project moving forward."

Later, Michael reflected on how different this response felt from his typical patterns. His punitive parent voice didn't attack him for making mistakes. His vulnerable child didn't feel devastated by criticism. His overcompensator mode didn't take over the entire meeting to prove his worth. Instead, some newer part of himself—what he was learning to call his healthy adult—had responded with wisdom, self-compassion, and appropriate confidence.

The healthy adult mode represents the integration of all the healing work we've explored throughout this book. Unlike child modes (which carry authentic emotions) or coping modes (which protect against perceived threats), the healthy adult operates from a place of wisdom, self-compassion, and realistic assessment of current circumstances rather than automatic reactions based on childhood learning.

## Characteristics of the Healthy Adult Mode

The healthy adult mode encompasses the mature psychological functioning that trauma often disrupts during development. This mode represents what optimal adult functioning looks like when it's not constrained by schemas, driven by survival responses, or controlled by internalized critical voices.

**Emotional regulation** in healthy adult mode means experiencing the full range of human emotions without being overwhelmed or controlled by them. The healthy adult can feel angry without becoming destructive, sad without falling into despair, anxious without being paralyzed, and joyful without feeling guilty or expecting it to end badly. Emotions become information and motivation rather than overwhelming experiences that require suppression or create chaos.

Consider how Jennifer's healthy adult learned to respond to relationship conflicts differently than her schema-driven patterns. Previously, disagreements with her partner would trigger her abandonment fears (vulnerable child mode), leading to either desperate attempts to fix the conflict immediately (compliant surrenderer mode) or preemptive withdrawal to protect against rejection (detached protector mode).

As Jennifer's healthy adult developed, she could recognize when her partner needed space to process disagreements rather than interpreting this as evidence of impending abandonment. She could express her own feelings and needs clearly while respecting his different processing style. Most importantly, she could tolerate the temporary discomfort of unresolved conflict without either suppressing her authentic responses or creating drama to force immediate resolution.

**Decision-making** from healthy adult mode involves gathering relevant information, considering multiple options, accepting uncertainty about outcomes, and making choices based on current values and circumstances rather than fear, shame, or automatic patterns from childhood.

David's healthy adult learned to make career decisions based on what genuinely interested and motivated him rather than what would prove his worth to others or avoid potential criticism. When considering a job change, his healthy adult could weigh factors like growth opportunities, work-life balance, and alignment with his values rather than just choosing the option that felt safest or most impressive to others.

**Problem-solving** in healthy adult mode focuses on practical solutions rather than self-attack, catastrophic thinking, or avoidance. When challenges arise, the healthy adult asks "What can I learn from this?" and "How can I handle this effectively?" rather than "Why does this always happen to me?" or "I should have prevented this."

**Boundary setting** from healthy adult mode involves clear, respectful communication about limits and needs without aggression, passive-aggression, or automatic accommodation of others' demands. The healthy adult can say no to requests that would be overwhelming while saying yes to opportunities that align with values and capacity.

**Self-compassion** represents perhaps the most distinctive feature of healthy adult functioning. This mode treats mistakes as learning opportunities, struggles as normal parts of human experience, and limitations as information rather than evidence of personal inadequacy. The healthy adult internal voice sounds like a wise, caring mentor rather than a harsh critic or demanding taskmaster.

**Developing Self-Compassion and Wisdom**

Self-compassion often feels foreign to trauma survivors because their developmental experiences taught them that self-criticism was necessary for motivation, protection, or maintaining relationships. Learning to treat yourself with basic kindness while maintaining appropriate responsibility and growth orientation requires both conceptual understanding and practical experience.

**Self-kindness** involves speaking to yourself with the same care you would offer a good friend facing similar challenges. This doesn't mean avoiding responsibility or making excuses for harmful behavior—it means addressing mistakes and difficulties without character assassination or catastrophic predictions.

**Common humanity** recognition helps you understand that struggles, mistakes, and limitations are normal parts of human experience rather than evidence of personal inadequacy. This perspective reduces the isolation and shame that often accompany difficulties and connects you to the broader human experience of learning and growing.

**Mindful acceptance** of difficult emotions and experiences allows them to be present without overwhelming you or requiring immediate action. The healthy adult can tolerate uncertainty, disappointment, and discomfort while maintaining perspective about their temporary nature and workable solutions.

The development of wisdom involves integrating emotional awareness with practical intelligence, personal values with consideration for others, and acceptance of current reality with motivation for appropriate change. Wisdom recognizes that most situations are more complex than they initially appear and that effective responses often require patience, perspective, and willingness to learn.

**Case Study: Michael's Emergence of Healthy Adult Functioning**

Michael's journey toward healthy adult functioning illustrates how integration of schema healing work creates new possibilities for responding to life challenges with wisdom and self-compassion rather than automatic trauma reactions.

**Starting Point and Trauma Patterns** Michael entered therapy at age thirty-eight following a workplace conflict that had triggered his familiar pattern of shame, self-attack, and emotional withdrawal. His schemas included defectiveness (believing he was fundamentally flawed), failure (expecting to fail at important tasks), and emotional inhibition (suppressing vulnerable feelings to avoid rejection).

These patterns had been reinforced by childhood experiences with a father who criticized constantly and a mother who was emotionally unavailable due to her own depression and anxiety. Michael learned that mistakes were evidence of personal inadequacy, that emotional expression was dangerous, and that safety required constant vigilance about potential criticism or rejection.

Michael's coping strategies included overcompensation (working excessively to prove his worth) and detached protector (emotional numbing to avoid vulnerability). While these strategies helped him achieve professional success, they also created chronic stress, relationship difficulties, and a persistent sense of emptiness despite external accomplishments.

**Schema Healing Foundation** Michael's healing work began with recognizing and challenging his core schemas through cognitive, experiential, and behavioral interventions. He learned to distinguish between his punitive parent voice ("You're incompetent and everyone knows it") and realistic assessment of his performance and areas for growth.

He practiced expressing vulnerable emotions in safe relationships, starting with his therapist and gradually extending to close friends and eventually romantic partners. This emotional expression work helped Michael access his vulnerable and angry child modes rather than automatically suppressing feelings that might provide important information.

Michael also worked on reducing his overcompensator mode by practicing "strategic imperfection"—deliberately doing some tasks at "good enough" levels rather than demanding excellence in every area of life. This helped him discover that his worth wasn't dependent on perfect performance and that most people didn't expect or require the impossible standards he placed on himself.

**Emergence of Healthy Adult Responses** As Michael's schema intensity decreased and his child modes became more accessible, space emerged for healthy adult functioning that wasn't driven by trauma patterns or protective strategies. This development happened gradually over eighteen months of conscious healing work.

In work situations, Michael's healthy adult could assess feedback objectively rather than interpreting all criticism as evidence of his inadequacy. He could acknowledge mistakes without catastrophic shame, ask for help when needed without feeling incompetent, and set appropriate boundaries around workload without guilt about not doing enough.

In relationships, Michael's healthy adult could express needs and feelings directly rather than withdrawing or overcompensating. He could tolerate conflict and disagreement without interpreting them as rejection, and he could offer support to others without automatically taking responsibility for their emotional well-being.

**Integration Challenges and Breakthroughs** Michael's healthy adult development wasn't linear or consistent. During times of stress, illness, or major life changes, his old patterns would resurface, and he would temporarily revert to schema-driven responses. Learning to recognize these temporary setbacks as normal rather than evidence of failure became part of his healthy adult functioning.

The breakthrough Michael described at the beginning of this chapter represented a moment when his healthy adult was strong enough to respond to challenge without being overwhelmed by schema activation. He could access multiple perspectives (the criticism might be valid, but it wasn't catastrophic), maintain emotional regulation (feeling concerned but not devastated), and respond with appropriate action (addressing legitimate concerns while maintaining confidence).

**Ongoing Development and Integration** Two years into his healing work, Michael reported that his healthy adult had become his dominant mode in most situations rather than an occasional experience during particularly good days. He could recognize when schemas or coping modes were activated and consciously shift to healthy adult responses rather than being controlled by automatic patterns.

Most significantly, Michael's relationships had deepened because he could be authentic without being overwhelmed by vulnerability, successful without needing to prove his worth constantly, and present without needing to control outcomes or avoid potential disappointment.

## Professional Strategies for Healthy Adult Cultivation

Schema therapy approaches healthy adult development through interventions designed to integrate healing work across all modes while building capacity for wise, compassionate responses to current life circumstances.

### Mode Integration Techniques

**Mode awareness training** helps clients recognize which mode they're operating from moment to moment and develop conscious choice about how to respond to different situations. This awareness provides foundation for choosing healthy adult responses rather than automatically reacting from child modes or coping strategies.

**Mode dialogue techniques** facilitate communication between different internal parts so they can work together rather than in conflict. The healthy adult learns to comfort vulnerable child modes, set limits with critical parent voices, and redirect coping modes toward more flexible responses.

**Transitional support** helps clients move from other modes into healthy adult functioning when they recognize that their initial responses aren't serving the situation effectively. This might involve breathing techniques, grounding exercises, or internal dialogue that helps access wisdom and perspective.

## Wisdom and Discernment Development

**Values clarification** helps clients identify what matters most to them across different life areas so they can make decisions based on authentic priorities rather than fear, shame, or automatic patterns from childhood.

**Perspective-taking exercises** help clients consider multiple viewpoints about challenging situations rather than automatically assuming the worst or most catastrophic interpretations of events and others' behavior.

**Long-term thinking development** involves learning to consider how current choices align with long-term goals and values rather than just managing immediate emotions or reactions to stress.

## Self-Compassion and Emotional Regulation Skills

**Self-compassion practices** help clients develop internal voices that provide comfort and guidance during difficulties rather than criticism and attack. These practices require repetition because self-compassion often feels foreign initially.

**Distress tolerance techniques** help clients experience difficult emotions without being overwhelmed by them or needing to escape immediately. This capacity allows for wise decision-making even during challenging circumstances.

**Emotional granularity development** involves learning to identify and articulate specific emotions rather than experiencing general distress or emotional numbing. This emotional awareness provides information for healthy adult decision-making.

**Daily Practice Guide: Healthy Adult Decision-Making Framework**

This framework helps you approach daily decisions from healthy adult mode rather than automatic reactions based on schemas, child modes, or coping strategies. Use this structure for both small daily choices and major life decisions.

**Step 1: Mode Recognition and Grounding**

Before making decisions, pause and assess your current internal state:

**Mode awareness questions:**

- What am I feeling right now in my body and emotions?
- Which mode am I operating from—child, coping, parent, or healthy adult?
- What automatic reactions or patterns am I noticing?

**Grounding techniques:**

- Take three deep breaths and notice your physical environment
- Feel your feet on the ground and your body in the chair
- Remind yourself of your current age, location, and safety

**Step 2: Information Gathering and Perspective Taking**

Approach the decision with curiosity rather than anxiety or pressure:

**Relevant information collection:**

- What facts do I need to make this decision effectively?

- Who might have useful perspectives or experience to share?

- What are the realistic possible outcomes of different choices?

**Multiple perspective consideration:**

- How might this situation look to someone without my particular triggers or sensitivities?

- What would I advise a friend facing this same decision?

- What are the various ways this situation could be interpreted?

**Step 3: Values and Priorities Assessment**

Ground your decision in what matters most to you rather than fear or external expectations:

**Values clarification:**

- What values are most relevant to this decision?

- How do different options align with what's important to me?

- What kind of person do I want to be in this situation?

**Priority evaluation:**

- What are my most important priorities right now in life?

- How does this decision support or interfere with those priorities?

- What would I regret more—taking action or not taking action?

**Step 4: Wise Action and Self-Compassion**

Make decisions with appropriate confidence while maintaining flexibility and self-kindness:

**Decision implementation:**

- Choose the option that best aligns with your values and current information

- Accept that you may not have perfect information and that's normal

- Commit to learning from outcomes rather than demanding perfect results

**Self-compassion integration:**

- Treat yourself kindly regardless of how the decision turns out

- Remember that making mistakes is part of human experience and learning

- Focus on effort and intention rather than just outcomes

**Step 5: Learning and Adjustment**

Use decision outcomes as information for future choices rather than evidence of personal worth:

**Outcome assessment:**

- What went well with this decision and what might you do differently?

- What did you learn about yourself, the situation, or your decision-making process?

- How can you use this experience to make better decisions in the future?

**Pattern recognition:**

- Are there themes in your decision-making that warrant attention?

- What schemas or modes tend to interfere with your decision-making process?

- How can you strengthen your healthy adult functioning over time?

### The Integration of All Parts

The healthy adult mode doesn't replace other parts of yourself—it provides leadership and integration that allows all parts to contribute their wisdom while preventing any single mode from controlling your life completely. This integration creates a richness and authenticity that wasn't possible when trauma patterns dominated your responses to life challenges.

**Child modes** continue providing emotional authenticity, creativity, and capacity for joy and connection. The healthy adult ensures these parts receive appropriate care and expression while maintaining adult functioning and responsibility.

**Coping modes** remain available for situations that genuinely require protection, detachment, or strategic responses. The healthy adult can choose when these strategies serve current circumstances rather than using them automatically based on childhood learning.

**Critical parent voices** may still arise during stress, but the healthy adult can recognize them as trauma patterns rather than accurate assessments and respond with compassion rather than belief in their harsh messages.

The goal isn't perfection or constant healthy adult functioning—it's developing enough integration and flexibility to respond to life circumstances with wisdom, authenticity, and self-compassion most of the time while having tools for returning to healthy adult mode when other patterns temporarily take over.

This integration represents the ultimate goal of schema therapy: not the elimination of all trauma responses, but the development of conscious choice about how to respond to life circumstances. The same intelligence that created survival patterns during trauma can create patterns that support thriving once safety and healing have been established.

### The Culmination of Healing

The healthy adult mode represents more than just another coping strategy or therapeutic technique—it embodies the integration of all healing work into a way of being that honors both your survival strength and your growth potential. This mode demonstrates that trauma doesn't have to define your life forever, that patterns formed in childhood can change, and that wisdom and compassion can develop regardless of what you experienced in your past.

The journey toward healthy adult functioning requires patience because it represents a fundamentally different way of relating to yourself and the world than what trauma teaches. Learning to trust your own judgment, treat yourself with kindness, and respond to challenges with curiosity rather than fear takes time and supportive relationships that can model these healthier patterns.

Yet the development of healthy adult functioning creates possibilities that extend far beyond symptom relief or problem management. It opens space for authentic relationships, meaningful work, creative expression, and genuine life satisfaction that may have seemed impossible when survival patterns dominated your responses to daily challenges.

Most importantly, healthy adult functioning becomes a gift you offer not just to yourself but to everyone in your life. The same wisdom and compassion that guide your own healing become resources you can offer others who are struggling. The stability and authenticity you develop through healthy adult mode create safe spaces where others can begin their own healing journeys.

The ripple effects extend across generations. Children who grow up with parents operating from healthy adult mode learn emotional regulation, self-compassion, and wise decision-making as natural parts of human functioning rather than skills they need to develop later through therapy. Partners experience the safety and growth that come from relationships based on authenticity rather than trauma patterns. Communities benefit from members who can contribute their strengths without being controlled by their wounds.

The healthy adult mode represents not an end point but a foundation—a stable platform from which you can continue growing, learning, and adapting throughout your life. It provides the internal resources necessary for navigating whatever challenges or opportunities arise while maintaining connection to your authentic self and compassionate treatment of your human limitations.

This integration of healing demonstrates one of the most hopeful truths about human nature: our capacity for growth and change continues throughout life. The patterns that helped you survive can be transformed into patterns that help you thrive. The intelligence that adapted to trauma can create wisdom that serves your authentic life. The same heart that learned to protect itself can learn to open safely to connection and love.

**Essential Elements of Healthy Adult Integration**

- The healthy adult integrates all parts of yourself rather than replacing them with new patterns

- This mode combines emotional authenticity with practical wisdom and self-compassion

- Development requires patience because it represents fundamentally different ways of relating to yourself and others

- Healthy adult functioning creates possibilities for authentic relationships and genuine life satisfaction

- This integration becomes a gift that extends to others in your life and future generations

- The goal is conscious choice about responses rather than automatic reactions based on childhood patterns

- Healthy adult mode provides a stable foundation for continued growth and adaptation throughout life

# Chapter 13: Cognitive Techniques for Trauma Schemas

Rachel stared at the thought record in front of her, pen hovering over the page as she tried to capture the automatic thoughts that had been tormenting her for weeks. "I'm going to mess up this presentation and everyone will see that I'm a fraud," she wrote, then stopped. For the first time in her adult life, she was questioning a thought that had felt absolutely true for as long as she could remember. Her therapist had taught her to ask a simple but revolutionary question: "Is this thought helpful, and is it based on facts or feelings?"

This moment marked the beginning of Rachel's cognitive transformation—learning to recognize the difference between schema-driven thoughts and realistic assessments of actual situations. After thirty-two years of believing that her anxious predictions were accurate reflections of reality, Rachel was discovering that many of her most convincing thoughts were actually trauma responses disguised as logical conclusions.

Cognitive techniques for trauma schemas represent some of the most practical and immediately applicable tools in schema therapy. Unlike approaches that focus primarily on emotional processing or behavioral change, cognitive work teaches you to recognize and modify the thought patterns that maintain trauma responses long after the original danger has passed.

## Schema-Focused Cognitive Restructuring

Traditional cognitive therapy focuses on identifying and changing distorted thoughts in specific situations. Schema-focused cognitive restructuring goes deeper by addressing the fundamental beliefs and thought patterns that create distorted thinking across multiple life areas and situations.

**Schema identification** forms the foundation of cognitive work because you can't change thought patterns you don't recognize. Many schema-driven thoughts feel so natural and automatic that people experience them as objective reality rather than subjective interpretations influenced by past experiences.

Consider how Tom's emotional deprivation schema created thought patterns that filtered every relationship experience through the lens of inevitable disappointment. When friends didn't return calls immediately, Tom's automatic thought was "They don't really care about me." When romantic partners needed space, he thought "This is the beginning of the end." When colleagues didn't include him in lunch plans, he concluded "I'm not important to anyone here."

These thoughts felt completely logical to Tom because his emotional deprivation schema had been filtering relationship experiences for decades. He had extensive evidence to support his negative interpretations because the schema caused him to notice and remember confirming experiences while dismissing contradictory evidence.

**Historical analysis** helps connect current thought patterns to their origins in childhood experiences. This process reduces the power of schema-driven thoughts by revealing them as learned responses rather than accurate assessments of current reality.

Tom's emotional deprivation schema developed during years of emotional neglect from parents who were physically present but emotionally unavailable. His father worked excessive hours while his mother struggled with depression that made emotional engagement nearly impossible. Tom learned that emotional needs were burdens and that expecting care from others led to disappointment.

Understanding this history helped Tom recognize that his current negative interpretations of relationship experiences were based on childhood learning rather than adult relationship realities. His friends' delayed responses had nothing to do with their care for him, and his partners' need for space reflected healthy boundaries rather than rejection.

**Evidence examination** involves systematically evaluating whether schema-driven thoughts are supported by current facts or influenced by past experiences. This process teaches you to distinguish between realistic concerns and trauma-based fears that feel convincing but don't match present circumstances.

The technique requires examining both supporting and contradicting evidence for automatic thoughts. Tom learned to ask questions like: "What evidence supports the thought that my friend doesn't care about me?" and "What evidence contradicts this interpretation?" This balanced analysis helped him recognize that delayed responses usually reflected busy schedules rather than lack of caring.

### Historical Tests and Schema Flashcards

Historical testing represents one of schema therapy's most powerful cognitive techniques because it directly challenges the childhood conclusions that formed schema patterns. These conclusions often made sense given limited childhood understanding and information, but they become problematic when applied to adult situations with different dynamics and possibilities.

**The historical test process** involves examining early experiences that contributed to schema development and evaluating those conclusions with adult perspective and understanding. This isn't about changing what happened in childhood but about updating the meanings and predictions that childhood experiences created.

Sarah's abandonment schema formed when her father left the family unexpectedly when she was six years old. Her child mind concluded that people you love will leave without warning and that expressing needs pushes people away. These conclusions helped her make sense of a traumatic experience but created problems in adult relationships where expressing needs actually strengthened connections.

The historical test helped Sarah examine her childhood conclusions with adult understanding. Her father's departure wasn't caused by her being too needy or demanding—it resulted from his own struggles with addiction and inability to handle family responsibilities. The leaving wasn't about her worth or lovability but about his limitations and untreated problems.

**Schema flashcards** provide portable tools for challenging schema-driven thoughts when they arise in daily life. These cards contain reminders about realistic interpretations, evidence that contradicts schema predictions, and alternative responses to schema activation.

Sarah created flashcards that she could review when abandonment fears arose. One card reminded her: "Dad left because of his addiction problems, not because I was unlovable." Another card listed evidence that contradicted her abandonment fears: "My husband has stayed through difficult times. My friends have been consistent for years. People actually appreciate my emotional openness."

**Thought monitoring and replacement** involves recognizing schema-driven thoughts as they occur and practicing alternative interpretations that are more balanced and realistic. This process requires patience because schema thoughts often feel more convincing than balanced alternatives initially.

The practice involves catching automatic thoughts, identifying the schema that's driving them, and consciously generating alternative explanations that fit current circumstances better than childhood-based predictions. Sarah learned to replace "He's late because he's losing interest in me" with "He's late because traffic is heavy and he has a demanding job."

### Case Study: Rachel's Cognitive Transformation Journey

Rachel's path from schema-driven thinking to cognitive flexibility illustrates both the challenges and rewards of learning to question thoughts that have felt absolutely true for most of your life.

**Background and Schema Patterns** Rachel grew up in a family where academic and social achievement were the primary ways to earn attention and approval. Her parents, both successful professionals, consistently communicated that ordinary efforts weren't sufficient and that mistakes were evidence of not trying hard enough or lacking intelligence.

These experiences created schemas of defectiveness (believing she was fundamentally inadequate), failure (expecting to fail at important tasks), and unrelenting standards (demanding perfection from herself). Rachel's thought patterns reflected these schemas through constant self-criticism, catastrophic predictions about mistakes, and impossible standards for performance.

By her thirties, Rachel had achieved considerable external success as a marketing manager, but her internal experience was dominated by anxiety and self-doubt that no amount of achievement could quiet. Her thought patterns included: "If I make any mistakes, everyone will realize I don't belong here," "I need to work twice as hard as everyone else to prove I'm competent," and "Success is just luck—eventually I'll be exposed as incompetent."

**Initial Cognitive Work and Resistance** Rachel's introduction to cognitive techniques felt threatening initially because questioning her thoughts felt like losing the vigilance that she believed kept her safe from failure and rejection. Her perfectionist thoughts, while painful, also felt necessary for maintaining the high performance that had earned her professional success.

The work began with thought monitoring exercises where Rachel tracked her automatic thoughts throughout the day without trying to change them initially. This awareness-building phase helped Rachel recognize how frequently her thoughts were dominated by self-criticism and catastrophic predictions about potential failures.

Rachel discovered that her mind operated like a harsh supervisor who constantly pointed out potential problems and criticized her efforts. She realized that she rarely had encouraging or supportive thoughts about her capabilities, even when facing challenges that were well within her competence range.

**Evidence Examination and Historical Analysis** The breakthrough came when Rachel began examining evidence for her automatic thoughts rather than automatically accepting them as facts. She learned to ask questions like: "What concrete evidence supports the belief that I'm going to fail this presentation?" and "What evidence contradicts this prediction?"

This process revealed that Rachel's negative predictions rarely materialized. Her presentations were typically well-received, her projects usually succeeded, and her colleagues often sought her input and collaboration. The evidence contradicted her schema-driven thoughts, but her attention had been so focused on potential problems that she hadn't noticed the positive feedback and successful outcomes.

Historical analysis helped Rachel understand that her current perfectionist thoughts were based on childhood experiences with parents who focused on mistakes rather than successes. Her adult work environment actually appreciated her contributions and didn't expect the impossible standards her family had demanded.

**Developing Alternative Thought Patterns** Rachel learned to generate balanced thoughts that acknowledged both challenges and capabilities rather than focusing exclusively on potential failures. Instead of "I'm going to mess up this presentation," she practiced thinking "This presentation has some challenging aspects, and I have the skills and preparation to handle them effectively."

This cognitive reframing felt artificial initially because Rachel's schemas had trained her attention to focus on problems and ignore strengths. Developing balanced thinking required conscious practice and repetition until more realistic assessments became automatic responses to challenges.

Rachel created schema flashcards that reminded her of evidence contradicting her defectiveness schema: "I've successfully completed dozens of challenging projects," "My colleagues regularly ask for my input and advice," "My track record shows competence, not incompetence."

**Integration and Ongoing Practice** After eighteen months of consistent cognitive work, Rachel reported a significant reduction in anxiety and self-criticism. She could approach challenging projects with realistic assessment of difficulties rather than catastrophic predictions about failure. Most importantly, she could enjoy successes rather than immediately focusing on the next potential problem.

Rachel's cognitive transformation wasn't complete or permanent—during times of stress or major challenges, her old thought patterns would sometimes resurface. However, she had developed tools for recognizing schema-driven thoughts and could usually shift to more balanced perspectives rather than being controlled by perfectionist predictions.

**Professional Protocols for Cognitive Interventions**

Schema therapy provides structured approaches for implementing cognitive techniques that address the deep-rooted nature of trauma-based thought patterns while maintaining safety and preventing overwhelming clients with too much cognitive challenge too quickly.

## Assessment and Psychoeducation Phase

**Schema assessment protocols** help therapists identify which schemas are most active and problematic for individual clients. This assessment guides cognitive interventions by focusing on the thought patterns that cause the most distress and life interference.

**Psychoeducation about schema development** helps clients understand how childhood experiences created current thought patterns. This education reduces self-blame and creates hope that patterns formed through learning can be changed through new learning.

**Thought pattern recognition training** teaches clients to identify when they're experiencing schema-driven thoughts versus realistic assessments of current situations. This discrimination forms the foundation for all cognitive intervention work.

## Cognitive Restructuring Implementation

**Thought monitoring protocols** provide structured ways for clients to track automatic thoughts, identify triggering situations, and notice patterns in their thinking. This data collection phase prevents cognitive work from being based on assumptions rather than actual thought patterns.

**Evidence examination techniques** teach clients systematic approaches to evaluating their automatic thoughts rather than accepting them as facts. This includes examining both supporting and contradicting evidence while maintaining balance and avoiding excessive optimism that doesn't match reality.

**Historical analysis methods** help clients connect current thought patterns to their origins while maintaining appropriate boundaries around trauma processing. This work requires careful timing to ensure clients have adequate coping skills before examining childhood experiences.

### Advanced Cognitive Techniques

**Schema mode cognitive work** addresses the different thought patterns associated with child modes, coping modes, and dysfunctional parent modes. Each mode requires different cognitive approaches because they serve different functions and operate from different developmental stages.

**Behavioral experiment design** helps clients test schema-driven predictions against reality through carefully planned activities that provide evidence about actual outcomes versus feared predictions. These experiments are designed to be challenging but achievable to prevent overwhelming clients with too much risk.

**Relapse prevention planning** helps clients prepare for situations that are likely to trigger schema activation and develop advance plans for using cognitive techniques during difficult periods. This preparation prevents temporary setbacks from becoming major regression.

### Workbook Section: Cognitive Exercises and Worksheets

These exercises provide structured practice for developing cognitive flexibility and challenging schema-driven thought patterns. Use them consistently rather than only during crisis periods to build cognitive skills that become automatic responses to challenging situations.

**Daily Thought Monitoring Exercise**

Track your thoughts for one week using this structured format:

**Situation:** What was happening when the thought occurred? **Automatic Thought:** What exact thought went through your mind? **Emotion:** What emotions did you experience and how intense were they (1-10 scale)? **Schema Connection:** Which schema might be influencing this thought? **Evidence For:** What evidence supports this thought? **Evidence Against:** What evidence contradicts this thought? **Balanced Thought:** What would be a more balanced way to think about this situation? **Emotion After:** How do you feel after considering the balanced thought?

Complete this exercise without trying to change your thoughts initially—focus on building awareness of your automatic thought patterns and their connection to your emotions and behaviors.

**Schema Evidence Log**

Create a running list of evidence that contradicts your most problematic schemas:

**For Abandonment Schema:**

- List relationships that have remained stable over time

- Record instances when people returned after temporary absence

- Note times when expressing needs strengthened rather than damaged relationships

**For Defectiveness Schema:**

- Document compliments and positive feedback you've received

- Record accomplishments and successes in different life areas

- List people who seek your advice or company

**For Failure Schema:**

- Chronicle projects and goals you've completed successfully

- Note times when you've overcome obstacles or learned from setbacks

- Record instances when your efforts led to positive outcomes

Review this evidence regularly, especially when schema thoughts are activated, to provide concrete reminders that schema predictions don't match your actual life experiences.

**Historical Test Worksheet**

Choose one of your strongest schema-driven beliefs and examine its origins:

**Current Schema Belief:** What belief about yourself, others, or the world causes you the most problems?

**Childhood Origins:**

- What experiences contributed to developing this belief?

- How old were you when these experiences occurred?

- What information and resources did you have available then?

**Childhood Logic:**

- How did this belief make sense given your childhood circumstances?

- What was this belief protecting you from or helping you survive?

- What would have happened if you hadn't developed this belief?

**Adult Perspective:**

- What information do you have now that you didn't have as a child?

- How might an adult observer interpret those childhood experiences differently?

- What other explanations are possible for what happened?

**Current Relevance:**

- Do your current circumstances match the conditions where this belief developed?

- How does this belief help or hinder you in your current life?

- What would change if you believed something different about this area?

**Schema Flashcard Creation**

Develop portable reminders that challenge your schema-driven thoughts:

**Evidence Cards:** Create cards that list concrete evidence contradicting your schemas. Include specific examples, dates, and details that make the evidence feel real and convincing.

**Perspective Cards:** Write alternative ways to interpret situations that typically trigger your schemas. Include questions that help you consider multiple explanations rather than automatically accepting schema-driven interpretations.

**Coping Cards:** List specific cognitive techniques that work best for you during schema activation. Include step-by-step instructions for evidence examination, thought replacement, or grounding techniques.

**Support Cards:** Include reminders about people you can contact for reality testing when schema thoughts feel overwhelming. List specific questions you can ask trusted friends or family members to get balanced perspectives.

**Weekly Cognitive Review**

Every week, assess your progress with cognitive techniques:

**Pattern Recognition:** What schema-driven thought patterns did you notice this week? Are you becoming more aware of automatic thoughts as they occur?

**Technique Use:** Which cognitive techniques did you practice? What worked well and what felt difficult or ineffective?

**Evidence Collection:** What new evidence did you gather that contradicts your schemas? How convincing does this evidence feel compared to schema-driven thoughts?

**Progress Assessment:** Are your automatic thoughts becoming less frequent or intense? Can you shift to balanced thinking more quickly than before?

**Goal Setting:** What specific cognitive skills do you want to practice in the coming week? What situations might provide opportunities to use these techniques?

## The Foundation of Mental Freedom

Cognitive work with trauma schemas provides something remarkable: the discovery that your thoughts are not facts, that childhood conclusions can be updated with adult perspective, and that the internal critic isn't your authentic voice but a learned response that can be changed.

This cognitive freedom doesn't happen overnight or without effort. Schema-driven thoughts often feel more convincing than balanced alternatives because they've operated for years or decades and connect to deep emotional patterns. Learning to question thoughts that have felt absolutely true requires courage and consistent practice.

Yet the liberation that comes from cognitive flexibility extends far beyond symptom relief. When you can recognize schema activation and shift to realistic thinking, you become free to respond to current situations based on present circumstances rather than childhood fears and assumptions.

Most importantly, cognitive techniques provide tools you can use independently throughout your life. Unlike therapeutic interventions that require professional support, cognitive skills become part of your permanent mental toolkit, available whenever schema thoughts try to convince you that old fears match current realities.

The journey from automatic acceptance of schema thoughts to conscious evaluation of their accuracy represents a fundamental shift in your relationship with your own mind. Instead of being controlled by thoughts that feel true but don't serve your current life, you become the observer and evaluator of your mental patterns, free to choose thoughts that support your growth and well-being.

**Cognitive Mastery Fundamentals**

- Schema-driven thoughts feel true but often don't match current reality or circumstances

- Historical analysis reveals childhood origins of current thought patterns and reduces their power

- Evidence examination teaches discrimination between realistic concerns and trauma-based fears

- Thought monitoring builds awareness necessary for cognitive change and pattern recognition

- Balanced thinking acknowledges both challenges and capabilities rather than focusing on extremes

- Cognitive techniques require consistent practice to become automatic responses to challenging situations

- Mental freedom comes from recognizing thoughts as interpretations rather than facts

# Chapter 14: Experiential Techniques for Trauma Healing

Carlos closed his eyes and allowed himself to return to the memory he had spent twenty-five years trying to forget— eight-year-old Carlos hiding in his bedroom closet while his father screamed at his mother in the kitchen below. But this time, instead of feeling helpless and terrified, adult Carlos entered the memory as a protective presence. He opened the closet door, knelt down beside his frightened child self, and said the words that eight-year-old Carlos had desperately needed to hear: "You're safe now. This isn't your fault. I'm here to protect you, and I won't let anyone hurt you."

The tears that followed weren't the familiar tears of helplessness and terror Carlos remembered from childhood. These were tears of relief, healing, and the profound recognition that the wounded child inside him had finally received the protection and comfort he had always deserved. This imagery rescripting session marked a turning point in Carlos's healing journey—the moment when he discovered that traumatic memories could be transformed through compassionate intervention rather than just endured or suppressed.

Experiential techniques represent the heart of schema therapy's approach to trauma healing because they address the emotional and somatic aspects of trauma that cognitive work alone cannot reach. While cognitive techniques help you understand and change thought patterns, experiential methods help you feel and heal the emotional wounds that created those patterns originally.

## Imagery Rescripting and Empty Chair Dialogues

Imagery rescripting stands as one of schema therapy's most powerful tools for trauma healing because it allows you to revisit painful memories while providing the comfort, protection, or justice that wasn't available during the original experience. This technique doesn't change what happened but transforms your relationship to traumatic events by introducing adult perspective and resources into childhood memories.

**The rescripting process** involves entering traumatic memories through guided imagery while maintaining awareness that you're safe in the present moment. The adult self can then intervene in the memory to provide protection, comfort, or advocacy that the child needed but didn't receive.

Maria's imagery work focused on a memory of being criticized harshly by her mother in front of extended family during a holiday gathering when she was ten years old. The original memory involved feeling ashamed, humiliated, and completely alone while adults either joined the criticism or remained silent. In the rescripted version, adult Maria entered the memory to comfort her child self and confront her mother about the inappropriate public criticism.

"You don't get to talk to this child that way," adult Maria said to her mother in the imagery. "She's learning and growing, and she deserves patience and kindness, not humiliation in front of everyone." Then Maria turned to her child self and said, "You didn't deserve that treatment. You're a good kid who was just being a kid. I'm proud of you for trying new things, even when they don't work out perfectly."

This rescripting transformed Maria's relationship to the memory from one of shame and isolation to one of protection and understanding. The emotional charge of the original memory decreased significantly because the child no longer felt alone and helpless in the traumatic situation.

**Empty chair dialogues** provide another powerful experiential technique that allows you to have conversations with people who harmed you, protected you, or represent important aspects of your healing process. These dialogues help you express feelings that may have been suppressed for years and practice new responses to old relationship dynamics.

The technique involves imagining that someone important to your healing process is sitting in an empty chair across from you, then speaking directly to them about your experiences, feelings, and needs. This externalization makes it safer to express intense emotions because you maintain control over the interaction while still accessing authentic emotional responses.

James used empty chair work to express anger toward his father that he had suppressed since childhood. His father's alcoholism and emotional abuse had created lasting patterns of fear and people-pleasing that interfered with James's adult relationships. In the empty chair dialogue, James could finally say things like: "Your drinking scared me every day. I never knew if you'd be kind or violent. I was just a kid who needed a father who could stay sober and treat me with basic respect."

These expressions helped James access and process emotions that cognitive work alone couldn't address. The anger wasn't destructive or overwhelming—it was clarifying and healing because it validated his childhood experience and gave voice to feelings that had been silenced for decades.

**Safety Protocols for Experiential Work with Trauma**

Experiential techniques can be profoundly healing, but they also involve accessing painful emotions and memories that trauma survivors have often spent years avoiding. Safety protocols ensure that this work promotes healing rather than retraumatization.

**Grounding and stabilization** form the foundation of safe experiential work. Before accessing traumatic material, you need solid grounding in present-moment awareness and reliable techniques for managing emotional intensity when it arises.

Basic grounding techniques include focusing on your physical environment (noticing what you can see, hear, and touch), connecting with your breath in a steady rhythm, and reminding yourself of your current age, location, and safety. These techniques help you maintain awareness that you're safe in the present even while accessing painful memories from the past.

**Titrated exposure** means working with traumatic material in small, manageable doses rather than trying to process everything at once. This approach prevents overwhelming your nervous system while still allowing meaningful emotional processing to occur.

Instead of diving into the most traumatic memories immediately, experiential work typically begins with less intense experiences that allow you to practice the techniques and build confidence in your ability to manage difficult emotions. You might start with imagery work around minor disappointments or frustrations before addressing major trauma events.

**Dual awareness** involves maintaining connection to both the memory you're processing and your current safety simultaneously. This dual perspective prevents you from becoming completely absorbed in traumatic material while still allowing authentic emotional engagement with healing imagery.

Throughout experiential work, you're reminded that you're an adult in a safe place choosing to do healing work, even while you're also connecting with childhood experiences and emotions. This dual awareness provides an essential safety net that prevents retraumatization.

**Integration and aftercare** help you process experiential work and maintain emotional stability after intense sessions. This might involve journaling about insights that emerged, practicing self-care activities that help you feel grounded, or scheduling additional support if needed.

### Case Study: Carlos's Healing Through Imagery Work

Carlos's journey through imagery rescripting illustrates both the power and the gradual nature of experiential trauma healing when conducted with appropriate safety measures and therapeutic support.

**Background and Trauma History** Carlos grew up in a household dominated by domestic violence where his father's unpredictable rages created constant terror for the entire family. From ages six through fifteen, Carlos witnessed his father physically and emotionally abuse his mother while feeling completely helpless to protect her or himself.

The trauma created lasting patterns of hypervigilance, emotional numbing, and relationship avoidance that persisted into Carlos's adult life. He struggled with intimate relationships because emotional closeness triggered memories of helplessness and terror. He also carried enormous guilt about not being able to protect his mother during childhood.

Carlos had tried various forms of therapy over the years, including cognitive therapy and medication, but he continued feeling disconnected from his emotions and unable to form close relationships. The traumatic memories remained vivid and distressing despite his intellectual understanding that he hadn't been responsible for his family's dysfunction.

**Initial Experiential Work and Resistance** Carlos's introduction to imagery work felt terrifying because it involved deliberately accessing memories he had spent decades trying to avoid. His initial response was to intellectualize the process rather than allowing authentic emotional engagement with the memories.

The work began with basic grounding and relaxation exercises that helped Carlos learn to manage anxiety and emotional intensity. He practiced imagery work with neutral or positive memories before attempting to access traumatic material, building confidence in his ability to enter and exit imagery states safely.

Carlos also worked extensively on developing his healthy adult mode before attempting rescripting work. He needed to strengthen his sense of adult competence and protection before he could provide these qualities to his childhood self in traumatic memories.

**Memory Processing and Rescripting** The breakthrough came when Carlos worked with the memory described at the beginning of this chapter—hiding in his closet while listening to his parents fight. This memory carried particular intensity because it represented his helplessness and isolation during family violence.

In the original memory, eight-year-old Carlos felt terrified, alone, and responsible for somehow stopping the violence below. The rescripting process allowed adult Carlos to enter the memory as a protective, comforting presence who could provide the safety and understanding that hadn't been available originally.

Adult Carlos told his child self: "This isn't your fault. You're not responsible for stopping dad's behavior or protecting mom—that's the adults' job. You're just a kid, and your only job is to stay safe. I'm here now, and I won't let anyone hurt you."

This intervention transformed the emotional content of the memory from helpless terror to protected safety. The child Carlos no longer felt alone and responsible for family dynamics he couldn't control. The adult Carlos could provide the protection and perspective that had been missing during the original experience.

**Expanding the Rescripting Work** Over several months, Carlos worked with multiple traumatic memories using imagery rescripting. Each session built on previous work while addressing different aspects of his trauma experience. He rescripted memories where he felt helpless, guilty, terrified, and alone, providing comfort, protection, advocacy, and understanding to his childhood self.

One particularly powerful session involved adult Carlos confronting his father in a memory where his father was threatening his mother. Adult Carlos could say things that child Carlos had been unable to express: "You don't get to treat your family this way. Your drinking and anger are your problems, not ours. These are children who need protection, not targets for your rage."

These confrontational rescripts helped Carlos access and express anger that had been suppressed since childhood. The anger wasn't destructive—it was protective and clarifying, helping Carlos establish internal boundaries that had been missing during childhood.

**Integration and Life Changes** After eighteen months of experiential work combined with cognitive and behavioral interventions, Carlos reported significant changes in his emotional life and relationships. He could access his emotions without feeling overwhelmed, and he had developed capacity for intimate relationships that had been impossible previously.

Most significantly, Carlos's hypervigilance decreased dramatically because his nervous system had received the message that protection was available. The imagery work had provided his traumatized child parts with the safety they had been seeking through symptoms for decades.

**Professional Trauma-Informed Experiential Protocols**

Schema therapy has developed specific protocols for conducting experiential work safely with trauma survivors, recognizing that these techniques require specialized training and careful attention to trauma-related triggers and responses.

## Preparation and Assessment Protocols

**Trauma assessment** helps therapists understand the nature and severity of traumatic experiences before beginning experiential work. This assessment guides the pace and intensity of interventions while identifying potential triggers that require special attention.

**Stabilization phase protocols** ensure that clients have adequate emotional regulation skills and support systems before beginning intensive experiential work. This phase might involve several months of cognitive and behavioral work to build coping skills.

**Safety planning** helps clients develop specific strategies for managing emotional intensity that might arise during or after experiential sessions. This includes both in-session grounding techniques and self-care plans for between sessions.

## Intervention Implementation Protocols

**Graduated exposure protocols** outline systematic approaches to experiential work that begin with less threatening material and gradually progress to more intense trauma processing. This prevents overwhelming clients while ensuring meaningful therapeutic progress.

**Session structure guidelines** provide frameworks for conducting experiential sessions that include adequate preparation time, careful monitoring during imagery work, and sufficient integration time after intense processing.

**Therapist stance and intervention guidelines** help therapists maintain appropriate therapeutic boundaries while providing the emotional attunement and support necessary for safe trauma processing.

**Safety and Crisis Management Protocols**

**Dissociation recognition and intervention** helps therapists identify when clients become disconnected during experiential work and provides specific techniques for restoring present-moment awareness safely.

**Emotional overwhelm management** includes protocols for helping clients regulate intense emotions that might arise during trauma processing without stopping therapeutic progress or creating additional trauma.

**Between-session support planning** ensures that clients have adequate resources and coping strategies for managing any delayed reactions to experiential work that might occur after therapy sessions.

**Guided Exercises: Safe Imagery and Dialogue Techniques**

These exercises provide structured ways to practice experiential techniques safely while building skills that support deeper trauma healing work. Start with shorter, less intense exercises before attempting longer or more emotionally challenging imagery work.

**Basic Safe Place Imagery**

Create a mental sanctuary you can access whenever you need emotional safety and calm:

**Preparation:**

1. Find a comfortable, private space where you won't be interrupted

2. Sit in a comfortable position with your feet on the ground

3. Close your eyes or soften your gaze downward

4. Take several slow, deep breaths to center yourself

**Imagery Creation:**

1. Imagine a place where you feel completely safe and peaceful—this might be a real location or an imaginary space

2. Notice the visual details—colors, lighting, textures, and objects

3. Notice the sounds—might be silence, nature sounds, or gentle music

4. Notice any scents or physical sensations—fresh air, warmth, softness

5. Allow yourself to feel the safety and peace of this place

**Anchoring:**

1. While experiencing the peaceful feelings, place your hand on your heart or another comforting touch

2. Take several deep breaths while maintaining the peaceful imagery

3. Tell yourself "I am safe and at peace" or another affirming phrase

4. Practice returning to this place by closing your eyes and using your physical anchor

Use this safe place imagery whenever you feel overwhelmed, before beginning other experiential work, or as a daily practice for emotional regulation.

**Self-Compassion Dialogue Exercise**

Practice speaking to yourself with the kindness you would offer a good friend:

**Setup:**

1. Think of a recent situation where you made a mistake or faced a challenge

2. Notice the automatic thoughts and emotions that arise about this situation

3. Identify the tone of your internal voice—critical, supportive, neutral?

**Compassionate Dialogue:**

1. Imagine speaking to a beloved friend who faced this same situation

2. What tone would you use—harsh and critical or kind and understanding?

3. What words would you offer—support, perspective, encouragement?

4. Now direct these same words and tone toward yourself

5. Notice any resistance to self-kindness and gently persist with compassionate language

**Integration:**

1. How does it feel different to speak to yourself with kindness rather than criticism?

2. What changes when you treat your struggles with the same compassion you'd offer others?

3. Can you commit to practicing this compassionate internal dialogue daily?

**Protective Figure Imagery**

Create an internal sense of protection and advocacy that can support you during difficult times:

**Imagery Development:**

1. Imagine a figure who represents perfect protection and care—this might be a person, spiritual figure, or symbolic presence

2. This figure has unlimited ability to protect and comfort you

3. Notice how this protective presence looks, feels, and communicates

4. Feel the safety and strength that comes from their protection

**Dialogue Practice:**

1. Share with your protective figure any fears or concerns you're carrying

2. Allow them to respond with wisdom, comfort, and reassurance

3. Ask them what they want you to know about your safety and worth

4. Accept their protection and care without needing to earn or deserve it

**Daily Integration:**

1. Practice calling on this protective presence during stressful situations

2. Imagine their support when facing challenges or making difficult decisions

3. Allow their strength to supplement your own during overwhelming times

**The Gateway to Emotional Freedom**

Experiential techniques provide access to healing that goes beyond intellectual understanding or behavioral change—they address the emotional and somatic wounds that trauma creates while providing corrective experiences that update your nervous system's understanding of safety and protection.

This work requires courage because it involves deliberately accessing emotions and memories that you may have spent years avoiding. Yet the avoidance itself often becomes more painful than the healing process, creating lives that feel limited by invisible barriers and unexplained reactions to present-day situations.

The beauty of experiential healing lies in its ability to provide what was missing during traumatic experiences—comfort for pain, protection during vulnerability, advocacy during helplessness, and understanding during confusion. These corrective experiences don't erase what happened, but they transform your relationship to traumatic events from one of helpless victimization to one of empowered survival and healing.

Most importantly, experiential work develops your capacity to be present with difficult emotions without being overwhelmed by them. This emotional presence becomes a foundation for authentic relationships, creative expression, and genuine engagement with life's challenges and opportunities.

The journey through experiential healing represents a return to emotional authenticity—the ability to feel your feelings fully while maintaining perspective, to access your emotions as information and energy rather than threats to be avoided. This emotional freedom becomes one of trauma recovery's greatest gifts, opening possibilities for connection and aliveness that may have seemed impossible during survival mode.

**Experiential Healing Essentials**

- Imagery rescripting provides corrective experiences that transform relationships to traumatic memories

- Empty chair dialogues allow expression of emotions that may have been suppressed for years

- Safety protocols prevent retraumatization while allowing meaningful emotional processing

- Grounding techniques maintain present-moment awareness during intensive emotional work

- Experiential healing addresses emotional and somatic aspects of trauma that cognitive work cannot reach

- These techniques require gradual practice and professional support for complex trauma processing

- Emotional authenticity and presence form the foundation for genuine life engagement and satisfaction

# Chapter 15: The Therapeutic Relationship in Trauma Work

The moment that changed everything in Susan's therapy happened not during a planned intervention or breakthrough insight, but during a simple exchange that lasted less than thirty seconds. Susan had been describing her latest work crisis with her usual self-deprecating tone when her therapist gently interrupted: "I notice you're telling this story as if you're the villain, but I'm hearing about someone who worked incredibly hard under difficult circumstances. Can we slow down and acknowledge that?"

For Susan, who had spent forty-three years expecting criticism and judgment from authority figures, this gentle correction felt revolutionary. Here was someone in a position of power who wasn't looking for her flaws or demanding perfect performance. Instead, her therapist consistently noticed her strengths, validated her efforts, and responded to her struggles with curiosity rather than judgment.

This experience of being seen accurately and responded to with consistent warmth became the foundation for everything else that happened in Susan's healing process. The cognitive techniques, experiential work, and behavioral changes that followed were all possible because the therapeutic relationship had provided something Susan had never experienced: a consistently safe, attuned, and supportive connection with another person.

The therapeutic relationship in trauma work serves functions that go far beyond the delivery of techniques or interventions. For many trauma survivors, the therapy relationship represents their first experience of what healthy connection can feel like when it's not based on performance, caretaking, or fear of abandonment.

## Limited Reparenting as Central to Schema Therapy

Limited reparenting stands as one of schema therapy's most distinctive and powerful techniques because it addresses the developmental needs that weren't met during childhood while maintaining appropriate professional boundaries. This approach recognizes that trauma survivors often need corrective relational experiences, not just insight or skill-building.

**The concept of limited reparenting** involves the therapist providing specific types of care, guidance, and emotional responsiveness that clients missed during their developmental years. This isn't about becoming a substitute parent or crossing professional boundaries—it's about offering targeted relational experiences that help heal specific developmental wounds.

Consider how limited reparenting helped Marcus heal his emotional deprivation schema. Marcus had grown up with parents who were competent providers but emotionally unavailable. His father focused exclusively on practical matters while his mother managed household tasks with efficient detachment. Marcus learned that emotional needs were burdens and that sharing feelings made others uncomfortable.

Marcus's therapist provided limited reparenting by consistently showing interest in his emotional experiences, validating his feelings as normal and understandable, and expressing genuine care about his well-being. These responses were carefully calibrated—warm and caring without being overly personal, interested without being intrusive, and supportive without creating dependency.

**Selective responsiveness** means that therapists provide the specific types of parental functions that clients missed while avoiding responses that might recreate harmful dynamics. Each client's limited reparenting needs differ based on their particular developmental wounds and current life circumstances.

For clients with abandonment schemas, limited reparenting might involve consistent availability, reliable follow-through on commitments, and explicit reassurance that temporary separations (vacation breaks, session cancellations) don't mean rejection. The therapist demonstrates that people can remain connected even during physical separations.

For clients with emotional deprivation schemas, limited reparenting involves genuine interest in their inner world, validation of their emotional experiences, and appropriate sharing of the therapist's emotional responses to their stories. This shows that emotions are valuable information rather than burdens that push people away.

For clients with defectiveness schemas, limited reparenting includes seeing and reflecting their strengths, maintaining consistent positive regard despite their mistakes and struggles, and responding to their flaws with understanding rather than criticism or rejection.

**Boundary maintenance** ensures that limited reparenting serves healing rather than creating new problems or dependencies. The therapist maintains professional boundaries while providing corrective relational experiences that help clients develop internal resources for healthy relationships outside therapy.

This balance requires skill and training because it involves being more relationally engaged than traditional therapy models while maintaining appropriate professional limits. The therapist might share more emotional responsiveness than in cognitive therapy but less personal information than in friendship.

### Managing Therapeutic Boundaries Safely with Trauma Survivors

Trauma survivors often have complicated relationships with boundaries due to childhood experiences where boundaries were either too rigid (emotional neglect) or too permeable (abuse, enmeshment). Creating therapeutic relationships that model healthy boundaries becomes part of the healing process itself.

**Flexible but clear boundaries** help trauma survivors experience relationships where limits exist for protection rather than rejection. The therapist maintains consistent professional boundaries while adapting their style to meet clients' specific relational needs.

Jennifer's therapy illustrates this balance beautifully. Jennifer had grown up with a mother who alternated between emotional enmeshment (sharing inappropriate personal information and expecting Jennifer to manage her emotions) and harsh rejection (cutting off all communication when Jennifer didn't meet impossible expectations).

Jennifer's therapist maintained clear boundaries about personal disclosure, session scheduling, and contact between sessions while being emotionally warm and responsive during their work together. This consistency helped Jennifer experience relationships where care doesn't lead to enmeshment and limits don't mean rejection.

**Transparent communication** about boundaries helps trauma survivors understand that therapeutic limits serve their healing rather than the therapist's convenience or rejection of them. Many trauma survivors interpret any limits as evidence that they're too much, too needy, or fundamentally unacceptable.

When Jennifer's therapist needed to reschedule a session due to illness, she explained the situation clearly and offered an alternative time promptly. She also checked in about how the schedule change affected Jennifer emotionally, normalizing any disappointment or concern while maintaining the boundary about her own health needs.

**Boundary violations as learning opportunities** can help trauma survivors practice addressing relationship problems directly rather than automatically assuming they caused the problem or that the relationship is ending. Therapists are human and occasionally make mistakes that can become valuable material for relational healing.

When Jennifer's therapist forgot to return a phone call promptly, she acknowledged the oversight, apologized for any worry it caused, and explored how Jennifer had interpreted the delayed response. This interaction helped Jennifer learn that relationship ruptures can be repaired and that she could express disappointment without destroying the connection.

**Graduation of boundaries** involves gradually shifting responsibility for boundary maintenance from therapist to client as healing progresses. Early in treatment, therapists may need to provide more structure and limits. As clients develop healthy relationship skills, they can take more responsibility for communicating their needs and limits.

## Case Study: The Therapeutic Relationship That Changed Everything

Patricia's story illustrates how the therapeutic relationship itself becomes a healing agent that transforms not just symptoms but fundamental beliefs about safety, worth, and the possibility of authentic connection with others.

**Background and Relational Trauma History** Patricia entered therapy at age thirty-six following a series of relationship failures that left her feeling hopeless about ever finding lasting love. Her pattern involved choosing partners who were initially attentive but eventually became critical, controlling, or emotionally abusive.

Patricia's childhood had been marked by emotional abuse from a mother who was unpredictably critical and rejecting. Her mother's moods determined the family's emotional climate—periods of warmth and approval alternated with explosive criticism and emotional withdrawal that could last for days or weeks.

This history created schemas of abandonment, mistrust, and defectiveness that made healthy relationships feel impossible. Patricia expected people to leave when they truly knew her, anticipated criticism and judgment from those in authority, and believed that her authentic self was fundamentally unacceptable.

**Initial Therapeutic Relationship Challenges** Patricia's early therapy sessions were marked by hypervigilance about her therapist's reactions and automatic assumptions that criticism or rejection were imminent. She monitored her therapist's facial expressions for signs of boredom or disapproval, apologized frequently for taking up time, and often asked if she was being "too much" or "too difficult."

Her therapist recognized these patterns as trauma responses rather than accurate assessments of their therapeutic relationship. Instead of interpreting Patricia's hypervigilance as resistance or neediness, she understood it as intelligent adaptations to a childhood where emotional safety was unpredictable.

The work began with explicit discussions about how trauma affects relationships and acknowledgment that Patricia's vigilance made sense given her history. This normalization helped Patricia recognize her patterns without shame while creating space for new experiences that could challenge her expectations.

**Corrective Relational Experiences** The healing happened through thousands of small interactions that contradicted Patricia's schema-driven expectations. When Patricia made mistakes or struggled with difficult material, her therapist responded with curiosity and support rather than criticism. When Patricia expressed anger or disappointment, her therapist remained present and engaged rather than withdrawing or retaliating.

Most significantly, Patricia's therapist maintained consistent warmth and positive regard even when Patricia tested the relationship through late arrivals, forgotten homework, or provocative statements designed to trigger rejection. These tests weren't conscious manipulation—they were trauma responses checking whether this relationship would replicate familiar patterns of conditional love and inevitable abandonment.

Each time Patricia's therapist remained steady and caring despite these challenges, Patricia received evidence that contradicted her core beliefs about relationships. People could stay connected even when she wasn't perfect. Authority figures could remain supportive even when she expressed difficult emotions. Authentic expression could strengthen rather than destroy connections.

**Internalization and Integration** Over time, Patricia began internalizing her therapist's consistent support and developing what she called "an internal good therapist" who could provide encouragement and perspective during difficult times. This internalized support helped Patricia maintain self-compassion and realistic thinking even outside therapy sessions.

The therapeutic relationship had provided a template for healthy connection that Patricia could recognize and seek in other relationships. She learned what it felt like to be seen accurately, accepted completely, and supported consistently—experiences that helped her identify similar qualities in potential friends and romantic partners.

**Relationship Pattern Changes** After two years of therapy, Patricia's relationship patterns had changed dramatically. She was dating someone who treated her with consistent respect and kindness—a dynamic that would have felt boring and suspicious earlier in her life but now felt safe and nourishing.

Most importantly, Patricia had developed the internal resources to recognize and address relationship problems directly rather than automatically assuming she had caused them or that the relationship was ending. The therapeutic relationship had taught her that conflicts could be worked through, that mistakes could be forgiven, and that authentic connection was possible when both people committed to honest communication and mutual care.

## Professional Guidelines for Trauma-Informed Relationships

Working therapeutically with trauma survivors requires specialized training and ongoing consultation because the therapeutic relationship itself becomes a powerful intervention that can either promote healing or inadvertently recreate traumatic dynamics.

### Foundational Principles for Trauma-Informed Practice

**Safety as the primary foundation** means creating therapeutic environments where clients feel physically and emotionally safe to explore difficult material. This includes predictable scheduling, clear communication about boundaries, and consistent responsiveness to clients' safety concerns.

**Trustworthiness through transparency** involves clear communication about therapeutic processes, honest acknowledgment of therapist limitations, and follow-through on commitments. Trauma survivors often have heightened sensitivity to betrayal or deception, making transparency essential for building therapeutic trust.

**Choice and collaboration** help clients regain sense of agency that trauma often destroys. This includes involving clients in treatment planning, respecting their pacing preferences, and supporting their autonomy in making life decisions rather than directing their choices.

## Specific Relationship Management Strategies

**Attunement and responsiveness** involve carefully monitoring clients' emotional states and adjusting therapeutic interventions accordingly. This might mean slowing down when clients feel overwhelmed, providing extra support during difficult periods, or celebrating successes that clients might minimize.

**Rupture and repair processes** help clients learn that relationship problems can be worked through rather than leading inevitably to abandonment or rejection. When therapeutic ruptures occur (misunderstandings, schedule conflicts, therapist errors), they become opportunities to model healthy conflict resolution.

**Graduated intimacy** involves slowly building therapeutic closeness at a pace that feels safe for trauma survivors. Some clients need significant time to develop trust, while others might seek inappropriate closeness too quickly as a way to avoid deeper intimacy fears.

## Supervision and Training Requirements

**Ongoing consultation** becomes essential when working with complex trauma because therapeutic relationships with trauma survivors can activate therapists' own attachment patterns and trauma responses. Regular supervision helps maintain therapeutic boundaries while providing adequate support.

**Specialized training** in trauma-informed practice ensures that therapists understand how trauma affects relationship patterns and have skills for providing corrective relational experiences safely. This training goes beyond basic therapy techniques to include understanding of attachment, trauma responses, and boundary management.

**Personal therapy requirements** help therapists understand their own relational patterns and trauma responses so they don't inadvertently recreate harmful dynamics with clients. Therapists who have done their own healing work can provide more authentic and boundaried relationships.

### Client Guide: How to Evaluate and Work with Your Therapist

Finding and working with a therapist who can provide healing relationship experiences requires knowledge about what to look for and how to evaluate whether the therapeutic relationship is supporting your healing goals.

### Qualities to Look for in Trauma-Informed Therapists

**Specialized training and experience** with trauma and attachment issues ensures that your therapist understands how childhood experiences affect adult relationship patterns. Ask about their training in trauma therapy, schema therapy, or other approaches specifically designed for developmental trauma.

**Consistent warmth and empathy** should be evident from your first contact. While therapists shouldn't be overly personal or friendly, they should communicate genuine care about your well-being and consistent interest in your experiences and feelings.

**Flexibility within clear boundaries** allows the therapeutic relationship to meet your specific healing needs while maintaining appropriate professional limits. Your therapist should be able to adapt their approach to your needs while maintaining consistent boundaries about scheduling, contact, and personal disclosure.

**Red Flags in Therapeutic Relationships**

**Rigid adherence to techniques** without attention to your emotional responses suggests a therapist who prioritizes methods over relationship. Trauma healing requires flexible approaches that prioritize your safety and readiness over predetermined treatment protocols.

**Inconsistent availability or responsiveness** can recreate abandonment dynamics rather than healing them. While therapists need appropriate boundaries, they should be reliable about scheduling, returning calls within reasonable timeframes, and providing clear communication about availability.

**Judgment or criticism** about your struggles, choices, or trauma responses indicates a therapist who hasn't developed adequate understanding of trauma's effects. Effective trauma therapy involves consistent validation and normalization of trauma responses rather than pathologizing them.

**How to Communicate with Your Therapist About Relationship Issues**

**Express concerns directly** rather than assuming the relationship is damaged beyond repair. Most therapeutic relationship problems can be worked through if both people are willing to communicate honestly about their experiences and needs.

**Ask for clarification** about boundaries, therapeutic approaches, or responses that confuse you. Trauma survivors often assume they've done something wrong when they don't understand therapeutic decisions, but most therapists welcome questions about their reasoning.

**Request specific relationship needs** based on your trauma history and healing goals. If you need extra reassurance about scheduling consistency, more frequent check-ins about your emotional safety, or specific types of validation, most therapists can adapt their approach to meet these needs.

### Building Skills for Healthy Relationships Outside Therapy

**Practice expressing needs and concerns** in the therapeutic relationship as preparation for using these skills in other relationships. The therapy relationship provides a safe place to practice direct communication, boundary setting, and conflict resolution.

**Notice and discuss relationship patterns** that show up in therapy as ways to understand how these patterns might affect other relationships. Your reactions to therapeutic boundaries, your expectations about your therapist's responses, and your fears about therapeutic ruptures often mirror patterns in other relationships.

**Use therapeutic insights** to evaluate and improve other relationships in your life. The understanding you develop about healthy relationship dynamics through therapy can help you recognize and seek similar qualities in friendships, romantic partnerships, and family relationships.

### The Healing Power of Being Known

The therapeutic relationship in trauma work represents more than a treatment method—it becomes a corrective emotional experience that can literally rewire your nervous system's understanding of safety, connection, and your own worth. For many trauma survivors, therapy provides their first experience of unconditional positive regard, consistent emotional availability, and authentic interest in their inner world.

This relational healing doesn't happen quickly or without challenges. Trauma survivors often test therapeutic relationships through behaviors designed to trigger familiar rejection patterns. They may arrive late, forget homework, express anger inappropriately, or become overly dependent as ways of checking whether this relationship will replicate childhood dynamics.

The healing happens through the therapist's consistent, boundaried response to these tests—staying present without becoming overwhelmed, maintaining care without becoming enmeshed, and setting limits without becoming rejecting. These responses gradually convince the trauma survivor's nervous system that different types of relationships are possible.

Most importantly, the therapeutic relationship becomes a template that trauma survivors can use to recognize and create healthy connections outside therapy. Once you've experienced what it feels like to be seen accurately, accepted completely, and supported consistently, you develop internal sensors that can identify these qualities in potential friends, partners, and communities.

The ripple effects extend far beyond symptom relief or problem resolution. When trauma survivors learn to trust their own worth through experiencing unconditional positive regard, they become capable of extending similar acceptance to others. The healing they receive becomes healing they can offer, creating expanding circles of safety and connection that extend across generations and communities.

**Therapeutic Relationship Foundations**

- Limited reparenting provides corrective experiences that address specific developmental wounds

- Consistent boundaries model healthy limits that protect rather than reject

- Therapeutic ruptures become opportunities to practice conflict resolution and repair

- The relationship itself serves as a template for recognizing and creating healthy connections

- Safety, trustworthiness, and collaboration form the foundation for trauma-informed practice

- Therapist training and personal healing work ensure competent boundary management

- The therapeutic relationship becomes a source of internal strength that extends beyond therapy

# Chapter 16: Behavioral Pattern-Breaking

Jennifer stood in the grocery store checkout line, her heart racing as she watched the total climb higher than she'd budgeted for the week. Her automatic response kicked in immediately—the familiar urge to put items back, apologize to the cashier for taking too long, and later criticize herself harshly for poor planning. But this time, something different happened. Jennifer paused, took a breath, and chose a different response.

"It's okay," she said quietly to herself. "I can afford this extra twenty dollars, and grocery budgets are estimates, not laws." Instead of the usual spiral of self-attack and corrective action, Jennifer paid for her groceries with calm acceptance of the minor budget overrun. This small moment represented a major victory in Jennifer's ongoing work to change behavioral patterns that had been automatic for three decades.

The shift from automatic trauma responses to conscious choice-making doesn't happen through insight alone—it requires systematic practice with new behaviors in real-life situations. Behavioral pattern-breaking provides the bridge between understanding your trauma patterns and actually living differently when those patterns get triggered by daily life circumstances.

### Identifying and Interrupting Schema-Driven Behaviors

Schema-driven behaviors often feel so natural and automatic that people don't recognize them as trauma responses rather than personality traits or necessary life strategies. These behaviors made sense in childhood environments where they served protective functions, but they often create problems in adult situations that don't require the same survival responses.

**Recognition training** involves learning to identify when you're operating from schema-driven patterns versus responding authentically to current circumstances. This awareness provides the foundation for behavior change because you can't choose different responses to patterns you don't recognize.

Take Amanda's people-pleasing behaviors that stemmed from her subjugation schema. Amanda automatically said yes to requests even when she was overwhelmed, agreed with opinions she didn't share, and suppressed her own preferences to maintain harmony. These behaviors felt like natural kindness and consideration rather than trauma responses that prevented authentic relationships.

Amanda learned to recognize her people-pleasing pattern by paying attention to physical sensations (tight chest, tense shoulders) and emotional responses (resentment, exhaustion) that arose when she automatically accommodated others' requests. These body signals helped her identify moments when she was operating from her schema rather than conscious choice.

**Trigger identification** helps you understand the specific situations, emotions, and interpersonal dynamics that activate automatic schema behaviors. This knowledge allows you to prepare alternative responses for predictable challenging situations.

Amanda discovered that her people-pleasing behaviors were most likely to activate when she perceived tension or conflict in relationships, when she felt criticized or judged, or when others expressed strong emotions. Understanding these triggers helped Amanda prepare different responses rather than being caught off guard by automatic reactions.

**Pattern interruption techniques** provide specific methods for creating space between trigger situations and automatic responses. This space allows you to choose conscious responses rather than being controlled by habitual patterns.

Simple pattern interruption might involve taking three deep breaths before responding to requests, asking for time to consider decisions rather than answering immediately, or physically changing your position when you notice schema activation. These brief pauses create opportunities for conscious choice-making.

### Graduated Behavioral Experiments for Trauma Survivors

Behavioral experiments involve systematically testing whether your schema-driven fears and predictions match actual outcomes in current life circumstances. These experiments are designed to be challenging but manageable, providing evidence that contradicts schema predictions without overwhelming your nervous system.

**Hierarchy development** involves creating lists of behavioral challenges organized from least to most difficult. This graduation allows you to build confidence and skills through success with easier challenges before attempting more threatening situations.

Robert's hierarchy for challenging his failure schema started with low-risk experiments like trying a new restaurant without reading reviews first, progressed to medium-risk challenges like volunteering for a project at work, and culminated in high-risk experiments like applying for a promotion he wanted but felt unqualified for.

Starting with lower-risk experiments allowed Robert to experience success and learn that his catastrophic predictions about failure rarely materialized. These positive experiences built confidence for attempting more challenging behavioral changes that his schema had convinced him were impossible.

**Prediction testing** involves clearly articulating what your schemas predict will happen in specific situations, then systematically testing these predictions through behavioral experiments. This process helps distinguish between realistic concerns and trauma-based fears.

Before each experiment, Robert wrote down his failure schema predictions: "I'll embarrass myself," "Everyone will see that I'm incompetent," "I'll fail and everyone will think less of me." After each experiment, he recorded what actually happened, often discovering that his feared outcomes either didn't occur or were much less catastrophic than predicted.

**Safety planning** ensures that behavioral experiments promote learning and growth rather than creating additional trauma. This includes starting with manageable challenges, having support available during experiments, and planning self-care for after challenging situations.

Robert's safety planning included choosing supportive friends to try new activities with, scheduling behavioral experiments for times when he had energy and emotional resources available, and planning rewarding activities after challenging experiments regardless of their outcomes.

**Case Study: Jennifer's Behavioral Transformation**

Jennifer's journey from compulsive caretaking to conscious choice-making illustrates how systematic behavioral work can transform patterns that feel essential to safety and relationships.

**Background and Behavioral Patterns** Jennifer had spent thirty-five years operating from self-sacrifice and approval-seeking schemas that created compulsive caretaking behaviors. She automatically took responsibility for others' emotions, volunteered for extra work projects, managed family logistics, and suppressed her own needs to maintain others' comfort.

These behaviors had earned Jennifer a reputation as someone people could depend on, but they also created chronic exhaustion, resentment, and relationships based on her usefulness rather than mutual care. Jennifer feared that setting boundaries or expressing her own needs would result in rejection and abandonment.

Jennifer's behavioral patterns included saying yes to all requests regardless of her capacity, apologizing excessively for normal mistakes, working late to ensure perfect results, managing others' problems before addressing her own needs, and avoiding activities that were enjoyable but not productive.

**Behavioral Assessment and Awareness Building** Jennifer's behavior change work began with detailed tracking of her caretaking behaviors, the situations that triggered them, and their emotional and physical effects. This awareness-building phase helped Jennifer recognize how automatic these patterns had become.

Jennifer discovered that her caretaking behaviors increased during family gatherings, work deadline periods, and any time she perceived interpersonal tension. She also noticed that these behaviors left her feeling depleted and resentful, even though she genuinely wanted to help others.

The tracking helped Jennifer distinguish between chosen acts of kindness and compulsive caretaking driven by fear of rejection. This discrimination became essential for developing alternative responses that maintained her generous nature while protecting her well-being.

**Graduated Boundary Setting Experiments** Jennifer's behavioral experiments involved gradually practicing boundary setting in increasingly challenging situations. She started with low-stakes situations where rejection was unlikely and progressed to more important relationships where boundary setting felt riskier.

Her initial experiments included declining invitations to events she didn't want to attend, asking for help with household tasks instead of managing everything alone, and expressing preferences about restaurants and activities rather than automatically deferring to others' choices.

Medium-level experiments involved saying no to non-essential work projects when her schedule was full, expressing disagreement with opinions in group conversations, and asking friends for emotional support rather than only providing it.

High-level experiments included having direct conversations with family members about dividing holiday responsibilities, setting limits with colleagues who regularly asked for extra help, and expressing needs in her romantic relationship rather than focusing exclusively on her partner's needs.

**Outcome Tracking and Schema Challenge** Jennifer systematically tracked the outcomes of her boundary-setting experiments, often discovering that her worst fears didn't materialize. Most people responded positively to her increased directness and authenticity, and the few who reacted negatively to her boundaries revealed relationships based on her caretaking rather than genuine mutual care.

These positive outcomes provided evidence that contradicted Jennifer's core schema beliefs. People didn't abandon her when she expressed needs. Relationships didn't end when she set limits. In fact, many of her relationships improved as she became more authentic and less resentful.

**Integration and Lifestyle Changes** After eighteen months of systematic behavioral work, Jennifer had developed what she called "conscious kindness"—the ability to choose when and how to help others based on her values and capacity rather than automatic fear of rejection.

Jennifer's life became more balanced as she learned to include her own needs in decision-making. She maintained her naturally generous spirit while protecting her energy for activities and relationships that truly mattered to her. Most importantly, she had developed trust in her own judgment about when to give and when to receive care.

### Professional Behavioral Intervention Protocols

Schema therapy approaches behavioral change through systematic protocols that address the deep-rooted nature of trauma-driven behaviors while preventing overwhelming clients with too much change too quickly.

## Assessment and Motivation Enhancement

**Functional analysis** helps identify the purposes that problematic behaviors serve so that alternative behaviors can meet the same needs in healthier ways. This analysis prevents trying to eliminate behaviors without addressing their underlying functions.

**Motivation enhancement** involves helping clients recognize both the costs and benefits of current behavioral patterns while building motivation for change. Many schema-driven behaviors have some benefits (safety, predictability, others' approval) that need acknowledgment before change becomes appealing.

**Readiness assessment** ensures that clients have adequate emotional regulation skills and support systems before beginning intensive behavioral change work. Behavioral experiments can activate schemas intensely, requiring coping resources to manage the anxiety that often accompanies pattern breaking.

## Behavioral Experiment Design and Implementation

**Systematic desensitization** involves gradually exposing clients to increasingly challenging behavioral experiments while maintaining emotional safety. This prevents overwhelming anxiety while building confidence through manageable successes.

**Prediction testing protocols** provide structured ways for clients to examine their schema-driven expectations against actual outcomes. This systematic approach to reality testing helps distinguish between realistic concerns and trauma-based fears.

**Safety planning integration** ensures that behavioral experiments include adequate preparation, support during challenging situations, and self-care after intense experiences. This planning prevents behavioral work from creating additional trauma or overwhelming coping resources.

### Progress Monitoring and Adjustment

**Outcome tracking systems** help clients and therapists monitor the effects of behavioral changes on symptoms, relationships, and overall life satisfaction. This data guides decisions about pacing, intensity, and focus of behavioral interventions.

**Flexibility in experiment design** allows for adjusting behavioral challenges based on client responses and changing life circumstances. Rigid adherence to predetermined behavioral plans can recreate trauma dynamics rather than promoting healing.

**Integration planning** helps clients incorporate successful behavioral changes into their ongoing lifestyle rather than viewing experiments as temporary therapeutic exercises. This integration ensures that behavioral changes create lasting life improvements.

### Action Plan Templates: Step-by-Step Behavior Change Guides

These templates provide structured approaches for implementing behavioral changes that address specific schema patterns while maintaining emotional safety and building lasting change.

**Template 1: Boundary Setting for People-Pleasers**

**Week 1-2: Awareness Building**

- Track all instances of saying yes when you want to say no

- Notice physical sensations when requests activate people-pleasing responses

- Identify the thoughts and fears that drive automatic accommodation

- Practice saying "Let me think about it" instead of immediate yes responses

**Week 3-4: Low-Risk Practice**

- Decline one invitation per week to events you don't want to attend

- Express preferences about minor decisions (restaurants, movies, activities)

- Ask for small favors from safe people to practice receiving help

- Practice expressing mild disagreement about non-controversial topics

**Week 5-8: Medium-Risk Challenges**

- Say no to one work request per week when your schedule is full

- Express needs or concerns in one relationship conversation per week

247

- Ask for emotional support when facing personal challenges

- Set time limits on helping behaviors to prevent exhaustion

**Week 9-12: High-Risk Integration**

- Have direct conversations about recurring boundary issues

- Maintain boundaries despite others' disappointment or pressure

- Choose activities based on your interests rather than others' approval

- Practice asking for what you need in important relationships

**Template 2: Risk-Taking for Perfectionist Patterns**

**Week 1-2: Perfect Standard Recognition**

- Identify areas where you demand perfection from yourself

- Track time spent on perfectionist behaviors (excessive checking, revising)

- Notice anxiety that arises when considering "good enough" standards

- Practice completing minor tasks at 80% rather than 100% effort

**Week 3-4: Controlled Imperfection Practice**

- Submit work emails without excessive proofreading

- Leave house with minor appearance imperfections (mismatched socks, unstraightened hair)

- Try new activities where you'll be beginner-level rather than expert

- Express opinions without extensive research and preparation

### Week 5-8: Visible Risk-Taking

- Volunteer for challenging projects at work despite uncertainty about outcomes

- Share creative work or ideas before they feel perfectly polished

- Ask questions in group settings even when you're not sure they're "smart enough"

- Make decisions with incomplete information rather than endless research

### Week 9-12: Integrated Excellence

- Choose strategically where to invest perfectionist energy vs. accepting good enough

- Take on leadership roles that involve visible mistakes and learning

- Practice public speaking or other activities with high visibility and uncertainty

- Develop personal projects based on enjoyment rather than achievement

### Template 3: Emotional Expression for Inhibited Patterns

### Week 1-2: Emotion Recognition

- Practice identifying emotions throughout the day using feeling words

- Notice physical sensations associated with different emotional states

- Track situations where you automatically suppress emotional responses

- Practice expressing emotions privately through journaling or art

**Week 3-4: Safe Expression Practice**

- Share feelings with trusted friends in low-risk conversations

- Express appreciation and positive emotions more freely

- Practice saying "I feel..." statements instead of "I think..." statements

- Allow tears or laughter without immediately suppressing emotional responses

**Week 5-8: Vulnerable Expression**

- Share struggles or fears with supportive people rather than managing alone

- Express disappointment or hurt directly rather than withdrawing or becoming passive-aggressive

- Ask for comfort during difficult times instead of handling everything independently

- Share excitement and joy even when others might not understand your enthusiasm

## Week 9-12: Authentic Communication

- Express anger appropriately when boundaries are violated

- Share needs and wants directly in important relationships

- Communicate during conflict rather than avoiding or shutting down

- Practice emotional intimacy by sharing your inner world with trusted people

## The Bridge Between Understanding and Living

Behavioral pattern-breaking represents the crucial bridge between understanding your trauma patterns and actually living differently when life triggers those familiar responses. Knowledge alone—even deep emotional knowledge—rarely changes automatic behaviors that have been practiced for years or decades.

The systematic practice of new behaviors gradually rewires your nervous system's automatic responses while providing evidence that contradicts schema-driven fears and predictions. Each time you choose a conscious response rather than an automatic pattern, you strengthen new neural pathways while weakening old trauma responses.

This behavioral work requires patience and self-compassion because it often feels uncomfortable or "wrong" initially. Trauma-driven behaviors feel natural and safe because they've been practiced extensively, while new behaviors feel awkward and risky even when they're objectively healthier.

The rewards of behavioral change extend far beyond symptom relief or problem resolution. When you can choose responses based on current circumstances rather than childhood fears, you become free to create the life you actually want rather than the one your trauma patterns allow.

Most importantly, behavioral changes become gifts you offer to the people in your life. When you can express needs directly, set boundaries appropriately, take reasonable risks, and share emotions authentically, you create space for others to do the same. Your healing becomes a permission slip for others to live more authentically in their relationships with you.

The journey from automatic patterns to conscious choice-making represents one of trauma recovery's most practical and life-changing aspects. It transforms daily life from a series of trauma reactions into opportunities for growth, connection, and authentic self-expression.

**Behavioral Change Foundation Points**

- Schema-driven behaviors feel automatic and necessary but often create problems in current life circumstances

- Pattern recognition provides the foundation for behavior change by creating space between triggers and responses

- Graduated experiments build confidence through manageable successes before attempting more challenging changes

- Systematic prediction testing distinguishes between realistic concerns and trauma-based fears

- Safety planning ensures that behavioral changes promote growth rather than creating additional stress

- Consistent practice gradually rewires automatic responses while providing evidence that contradicts schema predictions

- Behavioral changes become gifts that create space for others to live more authentically in relationships

# Chapter 17: Integrating Schema Therapy with Other Trauma Treatments

Marcus sat in his therapist's office describing the strange but wonderful experience of finally feeling progress after years of struggling with traditional therapy approaches. "The EMDR helped me process the specific memories," he explained, "but I kept falling back into the same relationship patterns. Then we added the schema work, and suddenly I understood why those memories had such power over my whole life. Now the somatic work is helping my body learn that I'm actually safe."

Marcus's experience illustrates what many trauma survivors discover: no single therapeutic approach addresses all aspects of complex trauma's impact on mind, body, and relationships. The most effective healing often comes from thoughtful integration of multiple evidence-based treatments that work together to address trauma's multilayered effects.

Schema therapy's flexibility and theoretical breadth make it particularly well-suited for integration with other trauma treatments. Rather than competing with approaches like EMDR, somatic therapies, or cognitive-behavioral interventions, schema therapy provides a framework that can incorporate techniques from multiple modalities while maintaining focus on the deep pattern change that lasting recovery requires.

## Schema Therapy and EMDR Integration

Eye Movement Desensitization and Reprocessing (EMDR) and schema therapy complement each other beautifully because they address different but related aspects of trauma's impact. EMDR focuses on processing specific traumatic memories and reducing their emotional charge, while schema therapy addresses the broader patterns and beliefs that those memories helped create (46).

**EMDR's memory processing strengths** include helping clients work through specific traumatic incidents, reducing flashbacks and nightmares, and decreasing the emotional reactivity associated with traumatic memories. These benefits create a foundation that makes schema work more accessible because clients aren't overwhelmed by unprocessed trauma reactions.

Sarah's treatment illustrates this integration perfectly. Sarah had experienced childhood sexual abuse that created both specific traumatic memories and broader schemas of mistrust, defectiveness, and vulnerability. Her therapy began with EMDR to process the most disturbing memories, reducing their emotional intensity to manageable levels.

Once Sarah could think about her abuse history without being overwhelmed by trauma reactions, she could begin examining how those experiences had shaped her beliefs about herself, others, and relationships. The schema work helped her understand why she continued choosing partners who were emotionally unavailable and why she felt responsible for others' inappropriate behavior toward her.

**Schema therapy's pattern-change strengths** include addressing the core beliefs and coping strategies that trauma creates, working with ongoing relationship patterns, and helping clients develop healthier ways of relating to themselves and others. These changes prevent the return of symptoms that can occur when trauma processing isn't followed by pattern change work.

The integration typically follows a staged approach. Initial EMDR work focuses on the most distressing memories that create ongoing symptoms like flashbacks, panic attacks, or severe anxiety. This processing creates emotional stability that supports deeper schema work focusing on beliefs, patterns, and relationship dynamics.

**Timing considerations** become crucial for successful integration. Beginning schema work too early can overwhelm clients who are still triggered by unprocessed memories. Starting EMDR too late can miss opportunities to address traumatic memories while they're most accessible through schema activation.

Maria's treatment demonstrated excellent timing when her therapist introduced EMDR during a period when her abandonment schema was highly activated due to relationship stress. The schema activation had brought childhood abandonment memories to the surface, making them accessible for EMDR processing while the current relationship situation provided motivation for deeper pattern change work.

### Combining with Somatic Approaches for Trauma

Trauma affects the body as much as the mind, creating patterns of chronic tension, hypervigilance, and disconnection that cognitive and emotional work alone cannot fully address. Somatic approaches like Somatic

Experiencing, body-based mindfulness, and trauma-sensitive yoga complement schema therapy by addressing the physical aspects of trauma storage and recovery (47).

**Body-based trauma symptoms** often persist even after successful cognitive and emotional processing because trauma gets stored in the nervous system and muscle memory in ways that verbal processing cannot fully access. Clients may understand their patterns intellectually and even feel emotionally resolved about past events while still experiencing physical symptoms like chronic pain, digestive issues, or sleep disturbances.

James's integration of schema therapy with Somatic Experiencing addressed his emotional inhibition schema through both psychological and physical approaches. His childhood had required constant emotional suppression to avoid triggering his father's rage, creating both cognitive patterns of emotional suppression and physical patterns of chronic muscle tension and shallow breathing.

The schema work helped James understand how his emotional inhibition developed and why it no longer served his adult relationships. The somatic work helped his nervous system learn to tolerate emotional expression without triggering fight-or-flight responses that had been conditioned during childhood.

**Nervous system regulation** becomes a foundation for all other therapeutic work because trauma often dysregulates the autonomic nervous system in ways that interfere with learning and change. Somatic approaches teach clients how to recognize and influence their nervous system states, creating stability that supports other interventions.

James learned to recognize when his nervous system was moving into hypervigilance or shutdown states and developed techniques for returning to calm alertness. This regulation created space for schema work because he could stay present during emotional conversations rather than automatically disconnecting when feelings arose.

**Embodied change** involves learning new patterns not just cognitively but somatically, so that healthy responses feel natural rather than forced. Many trauma survivors can intellectually understand healthier patterns but struggle to implement them because their bodies still carry trauma responses that override conscious intentions.

The combination of schema and somatic work helped James develop embodied emotional expression where sharing feelings felt safe and natural rather than threatening. His body learned through repeated positive experiences that emotional expression could strengthen rather than damage relationships.

### Case Study: Multi-Modal Treatment Success Story

Amanda's healing journey demonstrates how thoughtful integration of multiple approaches can address complex trauma more effectively than any single modality alone. Her treatment included schema therapy, EMDR, somatic work, and brief cognitive-behavioral interventions, each addressing different aspects of her trauma presentation.

**Background and Complex Trauma Presentation** Amanda entered treatment at age twenty-nine following a workplace assault that had triggered a cascade of symptoms including panic attacks, depression, relationship difficulties, and physical problems. While the recent assault was the immediate trigger, assessment revealed a history of childhood emotional abuse and neglect that had created lasting vulnerability.

Amanda's schemas included abandonment (fear that people would leave), emotional deprivation (expectation that emotional needs wouldn't be met), defectiveness (belief that she was fundamentally flawed), and mistrust (expectation that others would hurt her). These patterns affected every aspect of her life, from work relationships to romantic partnerships to self-care behaviors.

The recent assault had reactivated these schemas while creating new trauma symptoms. Amanda was experiencing flashbacks and panic attacks related to the recent event while also struggling with relationship patterns and self-concept issues that predated the assault by decades.

**Phase 1: Stabilization and EMDR (Months 1-6)** Amanda's treatment began with stabilization work focusing on developing coping skills for managing panic attacks and building emotional regulation capacity. This phase included psychoeducation about trauma's effects, grounding techniques, and basic schema education to help Amanda understand her reactions.

EMDR processing began once Amanda had developed adequate coping skills and therapeutic trust. The initial EMDR work focused on the workplace assault memories, reducing their emotional intensity and eliminating the flashbacks that were interfering with her daily functioning.

This processing provided significant symptom relief and created emotional space for examining the deeper patterns that the assault had triggered. Amanda could think about the recent trauma without being overwhelmed, which made it possible to explore connections to her childhood experiences.

**Phase 2: Schema Therapy and Pattern Recognition (Months 6-18)** With the recent trauma processed, Amanda could begin examining the schema patterns that had made the assault so devastating and that continued creating problems in her relationships and self-perception. The schema work helped Amanda understand why the assault had confirmed her existing beliefs about being unsafe and unworthy of protection.

Amanda discovered that her emotional deprivation schema had led her to ignore warning signs about the colleague who assaulted her because she was grateful for any attention and didn't trust her own discomfort with his inappropriate behavior. Her defectiveness schema convinced her that the assault was somehow her fault, while her mistrust schema prevented her from seeking support afterward.

The schema work involved cognitive techniques to challenge these beliefs, experiential work to access and heal childhood wounds, and behavioral experiments to test new ways of relating to herself and others. Amanda learned to recognize schema activation and developed alternative responses based on current reality rather than childhood learning.

**Phase 3: Somatic Integration and Embodied Healing (Months 12-24)** While the EMDR and schema work had created significant cognitive and emotional progress, Amanda continued experiencing physical symptoms including chronic tension, digestive problems, and sleep difficulties. The somatic component addressed these symptoms while helping Amanda develop embodied sense of safety and empowerment.

The somatic work included body awareness exercises, breathwork, gentle movement, and nervous system regulation techniques. Amanda learned to recognize how trauma and schema activation showed up in her body and developed tools for returning to calm, grounded states.

This embodied work was particularly important for Amanda's recovery because her childhood had included not just emotional abuse but also physical intimidation and boundary violations. Her body carried memories of being unsafe that needed direct attention through somatic approaches.

**Phase 4: Integration and Relapse Prevention (Months 18-30)** The final phase focused on integrating insights and skills from all treatment modalities while building Amanda's capacity for ongoing growth and self-care. This included practicing her skills during challenging situations, developing support systems, and creating plans for managing future stressors.

Amanda's integrated healing showed up in multiple ways: she could handle work stress without panic attacks, she had developed a healthy romantic relationship based on mutual respect, she could set appropriate boundaries with family members, and she experienced her body as a source of strength rather than vulnerability.

**Long-term Outcomes and Integration** Three years after completing intensive treatment, Amanda reported sustained improvements across all areas of her life. The EMDR had eliminated trauma symptoms related to the assault. The schema work had changed her fundamental beliefs about herself and relationships. The somatic work had created lasting changes in how she experienced safety and empowerment in her body.

Most importantly, Amanda had developed an integrated approach to self-care that drew from all the modalities she had experienced. She used EMDR-based techniques for processing new difficult experiences, schema therapy tools for recognizing and changing old patterns, and somatic practices for maintaining nervous system regulation and embodied well-being.

### Professional Integration Guidelines

Successful integration of multiple trauma treatments requires careful planning, proper training, and ongoing coordination to ensure that different approaches complement rather than interfere with each other.

### Treatment Sequencing and Coordination

**Assessment-based treatment planning** helps determine which interventions to prioritize based on clients' specific presentations, trauma histories, and current symptoms. Some clients need stabilization before memory processing, while others benefit from immediate trauma-focused work.

**Phase-based treatment models** provide frameworks for coordinating different interventions across time rather than trying to implement everything simultaneously. This typically includes stabilization phases, trauma processing phases, and integration phases that can incorporate different modalities as appropriate.

**Communication between providers** becomes essential when clients are seeing multiple therapists or working with treatment teams. Clear communication about treatment goals, client progress, and potential interactions between interventions prevents conflicting approaches that could slow healing.

**Training and Competency Requirements**

**Multi-modal training** ensures that therapists have adequate knowledge of different approaches to integrate them safely and effectively. This doesn't require mastery of every modality but does require understanding how different approaches work and when they're indicated.

**Supervision and consultation** support therapists in making decisions about treatment integration, particularly for complex cases that don't fit standard protocols. Regular consultation helps prevent therapist bias toward familiar approaches at the expense of what clients actually need.

**Ongoing education** about trauma treatment developments helps therapists stay current with research about treatment integration and new approaches that might benefit their clients. The trauma treatment field continues developing rapidly, with new understanding of effective combinations emerging regularly.

**Safety and Ethical Considerations**

**Scope of practice adherence** ensures that therapists only provide interventions within their training and competency area while making appropriate referrals for services they cannot provide. Integration doesn't mean every therapist should attempt to provide every type of intervention.

**Informed consent** about integrated treatment approaches helps clients understand what to expect from different interventions and how they work together toward treatment goals. This includes discussion of potential risks and benefits of each approach.

**Cultural and individual adaptation** ensures that treatment integration considers clients' cultural backgrounds, personal preferences, and individual presentations rather than applying standard protocols regardless of client characteristics.

### Resource Guide: Finding Integrated Treatment Approaches

Locating therapists and programs that can provide integrated trauma treatment requires knowing what to look for and how to evaluate providers' qualifications and approaches.

### Identifying Qualified Providers

**Training credentials** provide the foundation for evaluating whether providers have adequate preparation for integrated trauma treatment. Look for specific training in trauma therapies, not just general mental health credentials.

Key training indicators include:

- Certification in specific trauma therapies (EMDR, Somatic Experiencing, schema therapy)
- Specialized trauma treatment training programs
- Ongoing continuing education in trauma-related topics

- Supervision or consultation relationships with trauma specialists

**Experience with complex trauma** matters more than general therapy experience because complex trauma requires specialized understanding of how childhood experiences affect adult functioning. Ask about providers' specific experience with developmental trauma, attachment issues, and personality-level change.

**Integration philosophy and experience** help determine whether providers can coordinate multiple approaches rather than just providing isolated techniques. Ask about their experience combining different trauma treatments and their approach to treatment planning for complex presentations.

**Treatment Program Evaluation**

**Program structure and coordination** indicate whether treatment programs can provide integrated care rather than disconnected services. Look for programs with clear communication between providers and coordinated treatment planning.

**Range of services available** shows whether programs can address multiple aspects of trauma recovery including individual therapy, group work, psychiatric consultation, and specialized services like EMDR or somatic therapy.

**Treatment philosophy and approach** help determine whether programs understand trauma's complex effects and can provide the comprehensive care that complex trauma requires. Avoid programs that promise quick fixes or focus exclusively on symptom management.

### Insurance and Financial Considerations

**Insurance coverage evaluation** helps determine what services your insurance will cover and what you may need to pay out-of-pocket. Many specialized trauma treatments have limited insurance coverage, requiring financial planning for treatment costs.

**Sliding scale and payment options** make specialized trauma treatment more accessible when insurance coverage is limited. Many qualified providers offer reduced fees based on income or payment plans that make treatment affordable.

**Treatment length and intensity planning** helps you prepare financially and logistically for the time investment that integrated trauma treatment typically requires. Complex trauma recovery often takes months or years, not weeks.

### The Power of Multiple Healing Pathways

Integration of multiple trauma treatment approaches recognizes a fundamental truth about complex trauma: it affects every aspect of human functioning—mind, body, emotions, relationships, and spirit. No single therapeutic approach can address all these effects completely, but thoughtful combination of evidence-based treatments can create healing that addresses trauma's full impact.

The key to successful integration lies not in combining as many approaches as possible but in thoughtfully selecting interventions that address specific aspects of each person's trauma presentation while working together toward comprehensive healing goals.

This individualized approach requires skilled clinical judgment, adequate training in multiple modalities, and ongoing assessment of how different interventions are affecting overall progress. It also requires patience from both clients and therapists because integrated treatment often takes longer than single-modality approaches but creates more lasting and comprehensive change.

Most importantly, successful integration recognizes that healing happens through relationship—both the therapeutic relationships that provide safety for healing work and the personal relationships that provide ongoing support for sustained recovery. The technical aspects of treatment integration serve the deeper goal of helping trauma survivors reclaim their capacity for authentic connection with themselves and others.

The future of trauma treatment lies increasingly in this direction of thoughtful integration that honors both the complexity of trauma's effects and the remarkable capacity of human beings to heal and grow when provided with appropriate support and evidence-based interventions.

**Integration Mastery Essentials**

- Multiple trauma treatments address different aspects of trauma's complex effects on mind and body

- EMDR and schema therapy complement each other by processing memories and changing patterns

- Somatic approaches address physical trauma storage that cognitive work cannot fully reach

- Successful integration requires careful sequencing and coordination between different modalities

- Treatment planning should be individualized based on specific trauma presentations and client needs

- Qualified providers need training in multiple approaches and experience with complex trauma

- Financial and logistical planning supports the extended timeframe that integrated treatment often requires

# Chapter 18: Group Schema Therapy for Complex Trauma

The silence in the room felt different this week—not the tense, uncomfortable silence of strangers afraid to be vulnerable, but the warm, contemplative quiet of people who had learned to trust each other with their deepest wounds. Elena looked around the circle at the seven other group members who had become her chosen family over the past eighteen months, each person representing a different part of her own healing journey.

"I never thought I'd say this," Elena began, her voice steady and clear, "but you all have become the family I always needed but never had. You've seen me at my absolute worst—having panic attacks, raging about my childhood, crying over relationships that didn't work—and you're still here. That's never happened to me before."

The murmurs of recognition and support that followed Elena's words captured something unique about group schema therapy for complex trauma. Individual therapy provides safety and specialized intervention, but group work offers something equally powerful: the experience of being known completely and accepted unconditionally by multiple people who understand your struggles from their own lived experience.

Group schema therapy creates a healing community where trauma survivors can experience corrective relationships that challenge their deepest beliefs about safety, belonging, and worth. In this carefully structured therapeutic environment, people learn that authentic connection is possible, that their struggles don't make them unacceptable, and that healing happens in relationship with others who share similar journeys.

**Group Processes in Schema Therapy**

Schema therapy groups operate differently from traditional therapy groups because they're specifically designed to address the schema patterns that complex trauma creates. The group structure, norms, and interventions all focus on creating experiences that challenge schemas while building the healthy relationship skills that trauma often disrupts.

**Limited reparenting in group settings** involves all group members learning to provide the emotional responses that trauma survivors missed during childhood. This isn't about group members becoming therapists for each other, but about learning to offer genuine care, appropriate support, and honest feedback in ways that promote healing rather than repeating harmful patterns.

Consider how Elena's abandonment schema was challenged through group experiences that contradicted her core belief that people leave when they truly know you. Over eighteen months, Elena shared her most shameful secrets, had conflict with other group members, struggled through difficult periods, and made mistakes that hurt others—yet the group consistently remained committed to her healing and growth.

These experiences provided evidence that relationships could survive authenticity, conflict, and imperfection. Elena's abandonment schema had been based on childhood experiences where emotional expression led to rejection, but the group showed her that expressing needs and feelings could actually strengthen connections when people were committed to mutual growth.

**Schema activation and healing in group context** creates opportunities for real-time recognition and intervention when trauma patterns emerge. Unlike individual therapy where schema activation gets discussed after the fact, group settings allow schemas to be activated and addressed as they're happening.

When Marcus's emotional deprivation schema got triggered by feeling overlooked during a group session, other members could respond immediately with the attention and validation his schema insisted wouldn't be available. This immediate corrective experience felt more convincing to his nervous system than any amount of cognitive work about his worth and lovability.

**Interpersonal learning** happens naturally in group settings as members practice new relationship skills with multiple people who have similar struggles. This practice generalizes to outside relationships more effectively than individual therapy skills because it involves actual relationship experiences rather than just preparation for them.

Group members learn to express needs directly rather than through schema-driven behaviors, set boundaries without damaging relationships, handle conflict constructively, and offer support without losing themselves in others' problems. These skills get practiced repeatedly in the safety of the group before being applied to more challenging outside relationships.

## Managing Complex Trauma in Group Settings

Working with complex trauma in group settings requires specialized knowledge about how trauma affects group dynamics and careful attention to creating safety that supports healing rather than triggering additional trauma responses.

**Safety creation becomes paramount** because complex trauma survivors often struggle with trust, boundaries, and emotional regulation in ways that can make group settings feel threatening rather than healing. The group structure must provide enough safety for vulnerability while maintaining enough challenge to promote growth.

Group safety gets created through clear agreements about confidentiality, consistent attendance expectations, guidelines for giving and receiving feedback, and explicit norms about supporting each other's healing rather than trying to fix or rescue each other.

Sarah's initial terror about joining a group reflected her mistrust schema's conviction that sharing vulnerable information would lead to judgment, betrayal, or attack. The group's consistent adherence to safety agreements and their genuine support during her early sharing experiences gradually convinced her nervous system that this group was different from the family environment where vulnerability had been dangerous.

**Trauma responses in group settings** can include dissociation during emotional intensity, hypervigilance about other members' reactions, emotional overwhelm when witnessing others' pain, or aggressive responses when feeling threatened or misunderstood. Group facilitators must recognize these responses as trauma reactions rather than resistance or difficult behavior.

Michael's detached protector mode would activate whenever group discussions became emotionally intense, causing him to mentally "leave" the group even while physically present. Rather than interpreting this as lack of engagement, the group learned to recognize Michael's dissociation and gently help him return to present-moment awareness.

**Pacing and intensity management** prevents group sessions from becoming overwhelming while ensuring that meaningful therapeutic work happens. This involves balancing emotional processing with stabilization, managing how much trauma content gets shared in single sessions, and ensuring that all members receive adequate attention and support.

The group learned to check in with each member's capacity for intensity at the beginning of sessions and adjust the focus accordingly. If someone was struggling with outside stressors or felt emotionally fragile, the group might focus on stabilization and support rather than intensive schema work.

### Case Study: The Healing Power of Group Witness

Rebecca's transformation through group schema therapy illustrates how being truly seen and accepted by multiple people can heal wounds that individual therapy alone cannot reach. Her journey demonstrates the unique power of group witness in challenging fundamental beliefs about worth, belonging, and the possibility of authentic connection.

**Background and Isolation Patterns** Rebecca entered group therapy after two years of individual schema therapy that had helped her understand her patterns but left her feeling isolated and different from others. Her childhood sexual abuse had created schemas of defectiveness, mistrust, and social isolation that convinced her she was fundamentally damaged and unfit for normal relationships.

Rebecca's adult life reflected these beliefs through patterns of social isolation, superficial relationships, and constant shame about her trauma history. She functioned well professionally but felt like she was performing normalcy rather than living authentically. The thought of sharing her real experiences with multiple people felt terrifying and impossible.

**Initial Group Resistance and Terror** Rebecca's first months in group were marked by minimal participation, hypervigilance about others' reactions, and constant urges to flee when discussions became emotionally intense. Her schemas convinced her that the group would reject her if they knew her real history and that other members' problems were more deserving of attention than her own.

The group's patience with Rebecca's gradual engagement provided her first evidence that relationships could accommodate different pacing and needs. Unlike her family of origin where emotional needs had to be expressed urgently or not at all, the group consistently created space for Rebecca to participate at her own pace.

**Gradual Vulnerability and Schema Challenge** Rebecca's breakthrough came during her eighth month in group when another member shared a sexual abuse history that resonated deeply with Rebecca's experience. For the first time, Rebecca heard someone describe feelings and struggles that matched her own internal experience exactly.

This moment of recognition gave Rebecca courage to share more of her own story, starting with small disclosures about shame and self-blame that other members received with understanding and validation rather than judgment or pity. Each positive response to her vulnerability contradicted her defectiveness schema's predictions about rejection and disgust.

**Group Response and Corrective Experiences** The group's response to Rebecca's full trauma disclosure provided healing experiences that challenged every aspect of her trauma-based beliefs. Instead of rejection, she received support. Instead of judgment, she received understanding. Instead of advice or attempts to fix her, she received witness and validation.

Most powerfully, other group members shared how Rebecca's courage in disclosing her trauma had helped them feel less alone with their own struggles. This response transformed Rebecca's shame-based belief that her trauma made her a burden into recognition that her healing journey could inspire and support others.

**Integration and Leadership Development** As Rebecca's schema patterns loosened, she began taking on informal leadership roles in the group—welcoming new members, offering support during difficult sessions, and sharing insights from her healing journey. These leadership experiences contradicted her social isolation schema by demonstrating that she had valuable contributions to make to community.

Rebecca's transformation over two years in group therapy was remarkable. She went from isolated, shame-based functioning to becoming a source of wisdom and support for others. The group had provided her with experiences of belonging, contribution, and authentic connection that individual therapy alone could not have created.

**Ongoing Relationships and Community** The relationships Rebecca formed in group therapy extended beyond the formal therapy structure into ongoing friendships and support systems. Several group members maintained connection after completing therapy, creating a chosen family based on mutual understanding and shared commitment to continued growth.

This ongoing community provided Rebecca with something she had never experienced: relationships based on complete knowledge and acceptance of her authentic self, including her trauma history and ongoing struggles. These relationships became a foundation for all her other connections, providing internal security that supported healthier choices in work, romance, and family relationships.

## Professional Group Facilitation Guidelines

Leading schema therapy groups for complex trauma requires specialized training and ongoing consultation because group dynamics can quickly become complex and potentially triggering for both members and facilitators.

## Group Composition and Preparation

**Member selection criteria** help create groups that can support each other's healing rather than triggering additional trauma. This includes assessing emotional regulation capacity, commitment to group process, and ability to maintain appropriate boundaries with other members.

**Pre-group preparation** involves individual sessions with potential group members to assess readiness, explain group processes, and address concerns about group participation. This preparation reduces anxiety and increases likelihood of successful group engagement.

**Group size and structure** affect the intimacy and safety possible in group settings. Smaller groups (6-8 members) allow for more individual attention and deeper relationships, while larger groups may provide more diverse perspectives but less individual focus.

### Facilitation Skills and Interventions

**Multi-person awareness** involves tracking each group member's emotional state, schema activation, and participation level while managing overall group process. This requires sophisticated clinical skills and ongoing training.

**Schema-focused interventions** adapt individual schema therapy techniques for group settings, including group imagery exercises, empty chair work with group witnesses, and behavioral experiments that involve other group members.

**Crisis intervention skills** become essential when group members experience trauma activation, dissociation, or emotional overwhelm during group sessions. Facilitators must be able to provide immediate support while maintaining group safety and process.

**Ethical and Boundary Considerations**

**Confidentiality management** in group settings requires clear agreements about what information can be shared outside group and careful attention to maintaining trust among members.

**Dual relationship prevention** helps ensure that therapeutic relationships don't become confused with social relationships in ways that could harm group process or individual healing.

**Cultural sensitivity** ensures that group norms and interventions consider members' diverse cultural backgrounds and don't inadvertently recreate systems of oppression or exclusion.

**Participation Guide: Making the Most of Group Therapy**

Getting the most benefit from group schema therapy requires understanding how to participate effectively while maintaining appropriate boundaries and self-care.

**Preparation for Group Participation**

**Readiness assessment** helps you determine if you're prepared for group therapy emotionally and practically. Group work requires ability to tolerate others' emotional intensity, capacity for self-regulation during triggering moments, and commitment to regular attendance.

**Goal setting** involves identifying what you hope to gain from group participation beyond general healing or feeling better. Specific goals might include learning to express needs directly, developing capacity for conflict resolution, or building authentic friendships.

**Practical preparation** includes arranging childcare, transportation, and work schedules to support consistent attendance, as well as preparing emotionally for the vulnerability that group participation requires.

**Effective Group Participation Strategies**

**Gradual vulnerability** involves sharing increasingly personal information as trust develops rather than either staying completely closed or overwhelming other members with too much intensity too quickly.

**Active listening skills** help you support other members' healing while learning from their experiences. This includes asking clarifying questions, reflecting what you hear, and offering support without trying to fix or rescue.

**Boundary maintenance** ensures that group relationships remain therapeutic rather than becoming enmeshed or codependent. This includes being helpful without taking responsibility for others' healing and receiving support without becoming dependent on group members.

**Challenges and Problem-Solving**

**Managing triggering content** involves developing skills for staying present when other members share traumatic material while taking care of your own emotional needs and limits.

**Handling conflict** with other group members provides opportunities to practice relationship skills in safe settings while learning that conflict doesn't have to damage relationships.

**Dealing with resistance** helps you work through urges to quit group when the work becomes challenging or when schemas get activated by group interactions.

## The Circle of Healing

Group schema therapy represents one of trauma recovery's most powerful resources because it addresses the relational nature of both trauma and healing. Trauma typically happens in relationship and creates lasting impacts on our capacity for connection, trust, and belonging. Healing these relational wounds requires more than individual insight—it requires corrective experiences in relationships that provide safety, acceptance, and mutual support.

The group setting creates a laboratory for practicing new relationship skills while receiving feedback and support from others who understand your struggles intimately. This shared understanding reduces shame and isolation while providing hope that healing is possible even from severe trauma.

Most importantly, group members often become resources for each other long after formal therapy ends. The relationships formed in group therapy can become foundations for ongoing growth, sources of support during future challenges, and communities where continued healing happens through mutual care and understanding.

The investment of time, energy, and vulnerability that group therapy requires pays dividends that extend far beyond symptom relief or problem resolution. It creates possibilities for authentic community, genuine belonging, and relationships based on complete acceptance of who you are rather than performance of who you think you should be.

For trauma survivors who have often felt fundamentally different from others, the group experience provides profound healing through the recognition that you are not alone, that your struggles make sense, and that healing happens in community with others who share your commitment to growth and authenticity.

**Group Therapy Success Elements**

- Group settings provide opportunities for healing relational wounds through corrective relationship experiences

- Multiple group members can challenge schemas more effectively than individual therapeutic relationships alone

- Real-time schema activation allows for immediate intervention and corrective responses

- Group witness reduces shame and isolation while providing validation for trauma experiences

- Practicing relationship skills with multiple people creates generalization to outside relationships

- Group safety requires clear agreements and skilled facilitation to prevent retraumatization

- Long-term benefits include ongoing community and support systems beyond formal therapy

# Chapter 19: Special Populations and Cultural Considerations

Dr. Maria Santos closed her eyes for a moment before responding to her client Antonio's question about whether she really understood what it meant to grow up undocumented in a family where showing emotions was seen as weakness. As a Latina therapist who had also navigated the complexities of cultural identity while pursuing mental health treatment, Maria knew that Antonio's question went far beyond therapeutic technique—it touched the heart of whether healing could happen across cultural differences and whether schema therapy could address trauma that was deeply intertwined with cultural oppression and marginalization.

"I understand that your schemas didn't develop in a vacuum," Maria responded carefully. "They formed in a context where machismo culture told you that vulnerability was weakness, where poverty meant that emotional needs felt like luxuries, and where being undocumented meant that trusting authority figures could literally be dangerous. Your emotional detachment wasn't just about family trauma—it was also about cultural survival."

This exchange illustrates one of mental health treatment's most important challenges: How do we adapt evidence-based therapies like schema therapy to serve people whose identities, experiences, and healing needs have been shaped by cultural factors that traditional therapy approaches often overlook or misunderstand?

Schema therapy's framework provides a foundation for culturally responsive treatment, but its implementation must be carefully adapted to honor the cultural contexts in which schemas develop and the cultural strengths that support healing and resilience.

## Cultural Adaptation of Schema Therapy

Schema therapy's focus on early experiences and their lasting impact makes cultural adaptation not just helpful but essential, because schemas always develop within specific cultural contexts that shape how children learn about relationships, emotions, success, and safety.

**Cultural schema formation** recognizes that what gets labeled as "early maladaptive schemas" in one culture might represent adaptive responses in another cultural context. The same emotional suppression that creates problems in individualistic cultures emphasizing self-expression might represent appropriate interdependence in collectivistic cultures valuing family harmony over individual needs.

Jose's story illustrates this complexity beautifully. Growing up in a traditional Mexican-American family, Jose learned to prioritize family needs over individual wants, defer to parental authority without question, and suppress personal emotions that might create family stress. These patterns served important functions within his cultural context— maintaining family cohesion, showing respect for elders, and preserving cultural values across generations.

However, these same patterns created problems when Jose began working in corporate environments that expected individual initiative, direct communication, and self-advocacy. His schema therapy needed to honor the cultural wisdom of his upbringing while helping him develop flexibility to function effectively in different cultural contexts.

**Strength-based cultural assessment** involves recognizing the adaptive value of patterns that might appear problematic when viewed through mainstream therapeutic lenses. Many behaviors that get pathologized in traditional therapy actually represent cultural strengths that have helped individuals and communities survive oppression, discrimination, and cultural displacement.

Ana's hypervigilance about authority figures made perfect sense when understood as a response to growing up in a family where interactions with police, immigration officials, and other authority figures carried genuine danger. Her "paranoid" attention to power dynamics wasn't pathological—it was intelligent adaptation to real threats that many people in her community faced.

**Integration of cultural healing practices** means incorporating indigenous healing traditions, spiritual practices, and community support systems that clients find meaningful rather than assuming that Western psychotherapy approaches will resonate with everyone's healing needs.

Maria's work with Indigenous clients often included traditional healing practices like smudging ceremonies, talking circles, and connection to land-based spiritual practices alongside schema therapy techniques. These cultural practices provided meaning and grounding that purely psychological interventions couldn't offer.

**Working with Specific Populations**

Different marginalized communities face unique combinations of trauma, discrimination, and cultural factors that require specialized understanding and adapted treatment approaches.

## LGBTQ+ Trauma and Schema Formation

LGBTQ+ individuals often develop schemas in response to family rejection, societal discrimination, and internalized homophobia or transphobia that create unique patterns requiring specialized understanding and intervention.

**Rejection sensitivity schemas** often develop when LGBTQ+ children experience actual or threatened rejection from family members based on their identity or expression. These schemas create hypervigilance about acceptance and belonging that can persist even in affirming environments.

Sam's abandonment schema developed not just from general family dysfunction but specifically from his parents' rejection when he came out as gay at sixteen. His schema therapy needed to address both the original family trauma and the ongoing impact of living in a society where his identity was often not accepted or celebrated.

**Internalized oppression** can create defectiveness schemas where LGBTQ+ individuals internalize negative societal messages about their identities. These schemas often require both individual work and connection to affirming community for effective healing.

**Identity integration challenges** mean that schema work with LGBTQ+ clients must address the complex process of developing authentic identity while navigating family, cultural, and societal expectations that may not support full self-expression.

## Military Veterans and Combat Trauma

Veterans often present with complex combinations of combat trauma, military cultural factors, and challenges transitioning to civilian life that require specialized understanding of military experience and culture.

**Military cultural schemas** include patterns around emotional suppression, hypervigilance, and mistrust that served survival functions in combat environments but create problems in civilian relationships and work settings.

Captain Rodriguez's emotional inhibition schema had served him well during multiple combat deployments where emotional expression could have compromised mission effectiveness and unit safety. His challenge involved learning when emotional expression was safe and appropriate in civilian contexts while maintaining the emotional regulation skills that had kept him alive during military service.

**Moral injury** represents a specific type of trauma that occurs when veterans witness or participate in actions that violate their moral beliefs, creating schemas of defectiveness, self-condemnation, and spiritual disconnection that require specialized intervention approaches.

**Transition difficulties** often involve identity confusion as veterans adapt from military culture that provided clear structure and purpose to civilian environments that may feel chaotic and meaningless. Schema work must address not just trauma symptoms but also the identity and meaning-making challenges that military transition creates.

**Survivors of Institutional Abuse**

People who experienced abuse in institutions like residential schools, foster care systems, or religious organizations face unique schema patterns related to betrayal by systems meant to provide care and protection.

**Systemic betrayal trauma** creates complex mistrust schemas that extend beyond individual relationships to include distrust of institutions, authority figures, and helping systems—including therapy itself.

Margaret's experience in residential schools had created profound mistrust of anyone in authority positions, including therapists. Her schema work needed to proceed very slowly with careful attention to power dynamics and collaborative decision-making that honored her expertise about her own experience.

**Collective trauma patterns** affect entire communities when institutional abuse is widespread, creating shared schema patterns that require both individual and community-level healing approaches.

**Cultural disconnection** often results from institutional abuse that deliberately separated children from their cultural communities, creating additional identity and belonging issues that individual therapy alone cannot fully address.

**Case Studies: Diverse Healing Journeys**

These detailed examples illustrate how schema therapy adapts to serve people from different cultural backgrounds while honoring their unique experiences and healing needs.

**Case Study 1: Kenji's Integration of Japanese Cultural Values**

Kenji, a thirty-five-year-old Japanese-American software engineer, entered therapy struggling with anxiety and relationship difficulties that he traced to growing up in a family that emphasized honor, achievement, and emotional restraint as core values.

**Cultural Schema Development** Kenji's schemas developed within a cultural context that valued group harmony over individual expression, academic achievement as a measure of family honor, and emotional restraint as a sign of maturity and respect. His unrelenting standards schema reflected not just family dysfunction but also legitimate cultural values about excellence and dedication.

His emotional inhibition schema served important functions within his family system—showing respect for parents, maintaining family face in the community, and avoiding shame that could affect the entire family's reputation. These patterns helped him succeed academically and professionally while creating problems in intimate relationships where emotional expression was expected.

**Culturally Adapted Assessment** Rather than pathologizing Kenji's emotional restraint or perfectionist standards, his therapist explored how these patterns served cultural functions while also creating personal distress. The assessment included questions about cultural identity, immigration history, and the specific ways that Japanese cultural values had been transmitted in his family.

This exploration revealed that Kenji's schemas reflected an intensified version of legitimate cultural values rather than pure pathology. His family's immigration experience had created additional pressure to succeed as a way of proving their worth in American society, leading to more rigid application of cultural values than might have occurred in Japan.

**Integration Approach** Kenji's therapy focused on developing flexibility around cultural values rather than abandoning them entirely. He learned to distinguish between situations where emotional restraint was culturally appropriate and relationships where emotional expression would strengthen rather than threaten connections.

The work included helping Kenji develop what he called "cultural code-switching"—the ability to adapt his emotional expression and achievement orientation to different contexts while maintaining his core cultural identity and values.

**Outcome and Cultural Pride** Kenji's healing included developing pride in his cultural heritage while gaining flexibility to function effectively in different cultural contexts. He could maintain emotional restraint in professional settings where it served him well while expressing emotions more freely in intimate relationships where vulnerability strengthened connection.

### Case Study 2: Aisha's Healing from Religious Trauma

Aisha, a twenty-eight-year-old Black Muslim woman, sought therapy after leaving a fundamentalist religious community where she had experienced spiritual abuse and gender-based oppression that created complex shame and identity confusion.

**Religious Trauma Schema Formation** Aisha's schemas developed within a religious context that taught her that questioning authority was sinful, that women's worth depended on submission and modesty, and that her natural emotions and desires were evidence of spiritual corruption. Her subjugation schema reflected both religious teaching and cultural patterns that emphasized women's deference to male authority.

Her defectiveness schema included specifically religious elements—shame about spiritual inadequacy, fear of divine punishment, and beliefs that her struggles indicated lack of faith rather than human responses to difficult circumstances.

**Spiritual and Cultural Assessment** Aisha's assessment included exploration of her relationship to spirituality, her cultural identity as a Black woman, and the intersection of religious trauma with racial oppression she had experienced in both religious and secular contexts.

This assessment revealed that Aisha's healing needed to address religious trauma without dismissing the spiritual and cultural aspects of her identity that remained meaningful and supportive. She wanted to maintain connection to Islamic faith and Black cultural community while healing from the specific religious interpretations that had been used to justify abuse.

**Faith-Integrated Healing** Aisha's therapy included collaboration with progressive Islamic scholars who could provide alternative interpretations of religious texts that had been used to justify her oppression. Her healing process included reclaiming spiritual practices that felt nourishing while developing critical thinking skills about religious authority.

The work honored Aisha's desire to remain Muslim while helping her distinguish between universal spiritual principles and specific interpretations that had been harmful to her development and well-being.

**Community and Identity Integration** Aisha's healing included connecting with other Muslim women who had experienced similar struggles, providing community support for her journey of maintaining faith while rejecting harmful religious practices. This community connection helped her realize that her struggles were shared experiences rather than individual spiritual failures.

## Case Study 3: David's Recovery from Generational Military Trauma

David, a forty-two-year-old Native American veteran, presented with complex trauma that included combat experiences, historical trauma from his tribe's forced relocation, and family patterns of alcoholism and emotional unavailability that spanned multiple generations.

**Intersectional Trauma Assessment** David's assessment needed to address the intersection of personal trauma, combat experiences, and historical trauma that affected his entire community. His schemas reflected not just individual family dysfunction but also the ongoing effects of cultural genocide and systemic oppression.

His mistrust schema included realistic assessment of threats from government institutions that had historically harmed Native American communities, while his emotional deprivation schema reflected both family patterns and cultural suppression of traditional emotional expression and healing practices.

**Cultural and Traditional Healing Integration** David's therapy included connection to tribal elders and traditional healing practices alongside schema therapy techniques. His healing process incorporated sweat lodge ceremonies, talking circles, and connection to ancestral wisdom that provided cultural grounding for his recovery.

The integration honored David's identity as both a military veteran and a Native American man, recognizing that his healing needed to address both combat trauma and cultural disconnection that military service had created.

**Community and Generational Healing** David's recovery included taking on leadership roles in his tribal community and working with other Native American veterans who faced similar challenges. His healing became connected to broader community healing from historical trauma and ongoing oppression.

### Professional Cultural Competency Guidelines

Working effectively with diverse populations requires ongoing education, self-awareness, and commitment to adapting therapeutic approaches to serve clients' cultural backgrounds and healing needs.

### Cultural Self-Assessment for Therapists

**Personal cultural awareness** involves examining your own cultural background, biases, and assumptions about healing, relationships, and mental health. This self-awareness prevents imposing your cultural values on clients from different backgrounds.

**Privilege and oppression understanding** includes recognizing how systems of privilege and oppression affect both your perspective as a therapist and your clients' experiences of trauma and healing. This awareness shapes treatment planning and therapeutic relationship dynamics.

**Ongoing education commitment** means continually learning about different cultural communities, historical trauma patterns, and culturally responsive treatment approaches rather than assuming that general therapy training provides adequate cultural competence.

### Culturally Responsive Treatment Planning

**Cultural strength identification** involves recognizing and incorporating clients' cultural resources, healing traditions, and community supports rather than focusing exclusively on pathology and dysfunction.

**Historical context inclusion** means understanding how historical trauma, discrimination, and oppression have affected clients' families and communities across generations, shaping current schema patterns and healing needs.

**Community connection facilitation** includes helping clients maintain or rebuild connections to cultural communities that support their healing and identity development, recognizing that individual therapy alone may not address collective trauma patterns.

### Adaptation of Schema Therapy Techniques

**Language and metaphor adaptation** involves using cultural metaphors, stories, and language patterns that resonate with clients' cultural backgrounds rather than imposing Western psychological concepts that may not translate effectively.

**Family and community integration** means adapting individual-focused techniques to include family and community members in ways that honor clients' cultural values about collective versus individual healing.

**Spiritual and traditional practice inclusion** involves incorporating clients' spiritual beliefs and traditional healing practices into schema therapy work rather than viewing them as separate or conflicting approaches.

### Self-Advocacy Guide: Finding Culturally Responsive Treatment

Locating mental health providers who can offer culturally responsive schema therapy requires knowing what to look for and how to advocate for treatment that honors your cultural background and healing needs.

### Evaluating Cultural Competence in Providers

**Cultural background and training assessment** includes asking about providers' experience working with your cultural community, specific training in cultural competence, and understanding of historical trauma patterns that may affect your healing.

**Treatment approach flexibility** involves determining whether providers can adapt their techniques to honor your cultural values and healing traditions rather than expecting you to fit into predetermined treatment models.

**Community connections** include asking whether providers have relationships with cultural community leaders, traditional healers, or other resources that might support your healing process.

### Questions to Ask Potential Therapists

Key questions for evaluating cultural responsiveness include:

- What experience do you have working with people from my cultural background?

- How do you adapt schema therapy techniques for different cultural communities?

- Are you familiar with the historical trauma patterns that affect my community?

- How do you incorporate clients' spiritual beliefs and cultural practices into treatment?

- Can you provide references from other clients from my community who would recommend your services?

**Advocating for Culturally Responsive Treatment**

**Clear communication about cultural needs** includes explaining your cultural background, healing traditions, and specific concerns about how your identity might affect treatment planning and therapeutic relationship dynamics.

**Boundary setting around cultural respect** involves communicating what cultural practices and beliefs are non-negotiable for you and what adaptations you need from standard therapeutic approaches.

**Resource sharing** includes educating your therapist about your cultural community if they're unfamiliar with specific traditions, historical experiences, or current community issues that affect your healing.

**The Wisdom of Many Paths**

Cultural adaptation of schema therapy reflects a fundamental truth about healing: there are many pathways to recovery, and the most effective approaches honor both universal human needs for safety, connection, and growth while respecting the specific cultural contexts in which those needs are expressed and met.

The schemas we develop don't exist in cultural vacuums—they emerge from specific family, community, and historical contexts that shape their meaning and function. What appears as pathology through one cultural lens may represent strength, survival, or wisdom through another. Effective treatment requires therapists who can recognize these cultural differences while maintaining commitment to evidence-based practice.

The future of trauma treatment lies increasingly in this direction of cultural humility and responsiveness, recognizing that healing happens most effectively when it builds on clients' existing cultural strengths while addressing the specific ways that trauma has disrupted their capacity for well-being within their cultural contexts.

Most importantly, culturally responsive schema therapy creates possibilities for healing that honors the full complexity of clients' identities and experiences. When treatment can address both individual trauma patterns and the cultural contexts in which they developed, healing becomes more than symptom relief—it becomes reclamation of authentic cultural identity and community belonging that trauma may have disrupted.

This approach requires courage from both therapists and clients to move beyond one-size-fits-all treatment models toward collaborative healing processes that recognize the wisdom and strength present in all cultural traditions while addressing the specific ways that trauma has affected individual lives and communities.

The goal isn't to eliminate cultural differences or force everyone into mainstream therapeutic models, but to create healing approaches that honor diversity while providing effective intervention for trauma's universal effects on human capacity for safety, connection, and authentic self-expression.

**Cultural Adaptation Core Principles**

- Schemas develop within specific cultural contexts that shape their meaning and adaptive value

- Cultural strengths and healing traditions should be integrated rather than replaced by Western therapeutic approaches

- Different populations face unique trauma patterns that require specialized understanding and intervention

- Historical trauma and ongoing oppression affect schema formation across generations and communities

- Therapist cultural competence requires ongoing education and self-awareness about privilege and bias

- Clients need treatment approaches that honor their cultural identity while addressing individual trauma patterns

- Healing happens most effectively when it builds on existing cultural resources and community connections

## Chapter 20: Building a Life Beyond Trauma

The email arrived on a Tuesday morning in spring, five years after Jennifer had completed intensive schema therapy for complex trauma. Her former therapist had asked previous clients to share updates about their healing journeys, and Jennifer found herself staring at a blank screen, searching for words to describe a life that had become almost unrecognizable from the person who had first walked into therapy—anxious, exhausted, and convinced that her relationship patterns were simply who she was meant to be.

"I'm writing this from my kitchen table," Jennifer began typing, "while my partner makes breakfast and my daughter colors at the counter. Five years ago, I couldn't imagine a scene like this—not just having a family, but actually being present for the ordinary moments instead of constantly scanning for problems or managing everyone else's emotions. I wake up most mornings feeling curious about the day ahead rather than dreading what might go wrong."

Jennifer's story illustrates something profound about trauma recovery: healing doesn't just eliminate symptoms or solve immediate problems—it opens possibilities for creating lives that feel authentic, meaningful, and genuinely satisfying. The ultimate goal of schema therapy extends far beyond managing trauma responses to building capacity for the kind of life you actually want to live.

Building a life beyond trauma requires understanding that recovery isn't a destination but an ongoing process of growth, choice-making, and meaning creation that continues long after formal therapy ends. The skills, insights, and internal changes that schema therapy creates become foundations for continued development rather than final solutions to life's challenges.

**Post-Traumatic Growth and Schema Healing**

Post-traumatic growth represents one of psychology's most hopeful discoveries: the recognition that trauma can become a catalyst for positive changes that might not have occurred without the struggle through difficult experiences. This growth doesn't minimize trauma's pain or suggest that suffering is beneficial, but it acknowledges that humans have remarkable capacity to find meaning and strength through adversity (61).

**Schema healing as foundation for growth** creates the internal stability necessary for post-traumatic growth to occur. When schemas no longer control your responses to life challenges, you become free to choose how to interpret and respond to difficulties based on your current values and goals rather than childhood survival patterns.

Marcus's experience demonstrates this connection beautifully. His childhood emotional deprivation schema had convinced him that relationships were ultimately disappointing and that emotional needs were burdens others wouldn't willingly meet. These beliefs prevented him from forming close connections and left him feeling chronically isolated despite professional success.

Schema therapy helped Marcus challenge these beliefs through cognitive work, experiential healing, and behavioral experiments that provided evidence for different possibilities. As his emotional deprivation schema loosened its grip, Marcus discovered capacity for authentic relationships he hadn't known existed.

**Growth through meaning-making** involves developing new narratives about your life experiences that incorporate both trauma's impact and your strength in surviving and healing from it. This process transforms trauma from something that happened to you into something that contributed to who you've become.

Marcus learned to tell his story differently. Instead of "I'm someone who can't trust relationships because my parents were emotionally unavailable," his narrative became "I learned to be extremely self-reliant as a child, which helped me succeed professionally, and now I'm learning to balance independence with healthy connection."

**Expanded life vision** becomes possible when trauma responses no longer limit your choices about relationships, career, living situations, and personal growth. Many trauma survivors discover that they had unconsciously organized their entire lives around avoiding trigger situations rather than pursuing authentic goals.

Jennifer's schema healing allowed her to recognize that she had been choosing romantic partners based on their emotional unavailability because available partners triggered her abandonment fears. As her schemas healed, she could choose partners based on actual compatibility rather than familiar but problematic patterns.

## Maintaining Progress and Preventing Relapse

Long-term recovery from complex trauma requires ongoing attention to maintaining the gains that intensive therapy creates while continuing to grow and adapt as life circumstances change. This maintenance isn't about preventing all difficulties but about maintaining the flexibility and self-awareness that support healthy responses to inevitable challenges.

**Schema awareness as ongoing practice** involves recognizing when life stressors activate old patterns so you can respond consciously rather than automatically reverting to trauma responses. This awareness becomes a lifelong skill that protects against losing therapeutic gains during difficult periods.

Jennifer learned to recognize when work stress or relationship conflicts activated her abandonment schema, creating urges to either cling desperately or withdraw preemptively. Instead of being controlled by these urges, she could use them as information about her emotional state and implement coping strategies before the schema gained full control.

**Skill maintenance through regular practice** ensures that therapeutic tools remain accessible during stressful periods when you need them most. Just as physical fitness requires ongoing exercise rather than one-time training, psychological health requires regular practice of emotional regulation, cognitive flexibility, and relationship skills.

Jennifer maintained a weekly practice of schema flashcard review, monthly check-ins with her support system, and quarterly written assessments of her relationship patterns and life satisfaction. These practices helped her notice gradual changes in functioning before they became serious problems.

**Support system development** creates ongoing resources for reality testing, emotional support, and accountability that supplement but don't replace the internal resources that therapy develops. Healthy support systems include people who knew you before your healing and can appreciate the changes you've made.

Jennifer's support system included family members who understood her trauma history, friends who had supported her through therapy, and new relationships formed after her healing that were based on her authentic self rather than trauma-driven patterns. This diverse support network provided different types of assistance during various life challenges.

**Professional maintenance relationships** might include periodic therapy check-ins, participation in support groups, or consultation with helping professionals during major life transitions. These relationships provide professional perspective without creating dependence on external help for normal life functioning.

### Case Study: Five Years Later - Sustained Recovery

Jennifer's five-year follow-up illustrates how schema therapy creates lasting changes that continue developing long after formal treatment ends. Her story demonstrates both the stability of schema healing and the ongoing growth that becomes possible when trauma responses no longer control life choices.

**Background and Initial Presentation** Jennifer had entered therapy at age thirty-two following a pattern of failed relationships that consistently involved partners who were emotionally unavailable, critical, or abusive. Her schemas included abandonment (fear that people would leave), emotional deprivation (expectation that emotional needs wouldn't be met), and subjugation (suppressing own needs to avoid conflict).

These schemas had controlled every aspect of Jennifer's adult life. She chose romantic partners who confirmed her expectations of disappointment, maintained friendships based on her caretaking rather than mutual support, and pursued career paths that felt safe rather than meaningful. Her life looked stable from the outside but felt empty and inauthentic to her.

**Two-Year Post-Therapy Assessment** Two years after completing schema therapy, Jennifer had made significant changes that demonstrated genuine schema healing rather than just symptom management. She had ended her relationship with an emotionally abusive partner and was dating someone who treated her with consistent kindness and respect.

Her career had shifted from a stable but unfulfilling administrative job to freelance work in graphic design that felt more aligned with her authentic interests and talents. Most importantly, she could tolerate the uncertainty and occasional disappointments that came with more authentic living rather than organizing her life around avoiding all potential problems.

Jennifer's relationships had become more mutual and satisfying. She could express needs and concerns directly, maintain friendships based on genuine connection rather than one-sided caretaking, and handle conflicts constructively rather than automatically accommodating others' demands.

**Five-Year Sustained Recovery** Jennifer's five-year follow-up revealed continued growth and stability that demonstrated the lasting nature of deep schema change. She had married her partner from two years earlier and they had built a relationship based on genuine compatibility rather than trauma-driven attraction to unavailable people.

Her business had grown into a successful studio with several employees, requiring leadership and decision-making skills that her previous schemas would have made impossible. She could handle business challenges, employee conflicts, and financial uncertainties without reverting to abandonment fears or subjugation patterns.

Most significantly, Jennifer had become a mother—a role that had terrified her during early recovery because she feared repeating her own childhood experiences. Her schema healing had given her confidence that she could provide the emotional availability and consistent care that her own childhood had lacked.

**Ongoing Growth and Challenges** Jennifer's recovery wasn't a straight line of continuous improvement. She experienced normal life stresses including business challenges, parenting difficulties, marriage conflicts, and family health problems that temporarily activated old schema patterns.

The difference was her response to these challenges. Instead of being overwhelmed by schema activation or reverting to old survival patterns, Jennifer could recognize schema triggers, use coping skills to manage emotional intensity, and address problems constructively rather than just react from trauma responses.

Her continued growth included developing new capacities that hadn't been possible during survival mode—creative expression through her art, leadership skills through business management, and parenting abilities that broke intergenerational trauma patterns.

**Integration of Therapy Learning** Jennifer's life demonstrated genuine integration of schema therapy principles rather than just application of isolated techniques. She had internalized the healthy adult mode as her primary way of functioning, with child modes and coping modes available when appropriate but not controlling her choices.

Her relationship with herself had become characterized by self-compassion rather than criticism, realistic assessment rather than catastrophic thinking, and authentic expression rather than performance of acceptable roles. These internal changes created stability that supported all her external life improvements.

### Professional Discharge Planning and Follow-Up

Ending intensive schema therapy for complex trauma requires careful planning to ensure that clients have adequate resources and skills for maintaining therapeutic gains while continuing personal growth independently.

### Graduation Criteria and Readiness Assessment

**Functional improvement markers** include sustained changes in relationship patterns, emotional regulation capacity, and life functioning that demonstrate genuine schema change rather than just symptom management. Clients should show ability to handle normal life stresses without reverting to old patterns.

**Internal change indicators** involve shifts in self-perception, relationship expectations, and emotional responses that suggest deep pattern change rather than surface behavior modification. Clients should report feeling different internally, not just acting differently externally.

**Independence and resource development** means clients have developed internal coping resources and external support systems that can maintain their progress without ongoing therapeutic dependence. They should feel confident about handling future challenges independently while knowing when to seek appropriate help.

**Transition Planning and Resource Development**

**Gradual treatment tapering** involves slowly reducing session frequency over several months rather than ending therapy abruptly. This gradual transition allows clients to practice independence while maintaining therapeutic support during adjustment periods.

**Resource identification and connection** helps clients develop ongoing sources of support, growth opportunities, and professional consultation that supplement their internal resources. This might include support groups, continuing education, spiritual communities, or periodic therapy check-ins.

**Relapse prevention planning** involves identifying early warning signs of schema reactivation and developing specific plans for addressing temporary setbacks before they become major regression. Clients learn to distinguish between normal life difficulties and signs that additional help might be needed.

**Long-Term Outcome Monitoring**

**Follow-up assessment protocols** provide structured ways to evaluate long-term treatment effectiveness while offering support for continued growth. This might include annual questionnaires, periodic phone check-ins, or availability for consultation during major life transitions.

**Booster session availability** ensures that clients can access professional support during particularly challenging periods without needing to restart comprehensive treatment. Brief consultations can often prevent minor setbacks from becoming major problems.

**Continuing education about schema therapy** helps clients maintain understanding of their patterns and stay current with new developments in trauma treatment that might support their continued growth. This might include reading materials, workshop participation, or online resources.

### Life Planning Workbook: Creating Your Vision for the Future

Building a meaningful life beyond trauma requires intentional planning that incorporates both your healing gains and your authentic goals and values. This workbook section provides structured exercises for creating a vision of the life you want to build with your newly developed capacities.

### Values Clarification and Life Direction

**Personal values assessment** helps you identify what matters most to you based on your authentic self rather than trauma-driven survival priorities or external expectations about how you should live.

Complete this sentence for each life area: "What matters most to me about _____ is _____"

- Relationships and family
- Work and career
- Personal growth and learning
- Community and contribution
- Health and self-care
- Creativity and expression
- Spirituality and meaning
- Adventure and exploration

**Trauma pattern recognition** involves identifying how your old schemas might have limited your life choices so you can make conscious decisions about expanding into areas that previously felt impossible or dangerous.

Questions for reflection:

- What activities, relationships, or goals did you avoid because of schema fears?
- What patterns of playing small or choosing safety over authenticity do you recognize?
- What dreams or interests did you abandon because they felt too risky or vulnerable?
- How might your life look different if schema fears weren't controlling your choices?

**Future Visioning and Goal Setting**

**Five-year vision development** involves creating detailed, positive images of how you want your life to look and feel when you're living from your authentic self rather than trauma patterns.

Vision areas to consider:

- What kinds of relationships do you want to have?
- What work or contribution feels meaningful to you?
- How do you want to spend your time and energy?
- What kind of person do you want to become?
- What legacy do you want to create?

**Goal hierarchy creation** helps you identify specific, achievable steps toward your vision while maintaining flexibility for growth and change as you continue developing.

Categories for goal setting:

- Short-term goals (3-6 months): Immediate steps you can take
- Medium-term goals (1-2 years): Larger changes requiring sustained effort
- Long-term goals (3-5 years): Major life changes or achievements
- Ongoing practices: Daily or weekly habits supporting your vision

**Action Planning and Implementation**

**Obstacle identification and planning** involves recognizing potential challenges to your goals and developing strategies for handling them without abandoning your vision or reverting to old patterns.

Common obstacles to consider:

- Schema activation during stress or transition periods

- Relationship changes as you become more authentic

- Fear of success or visibility that trauma survivors often experience

- Financial or practical barriers to goal achievement

- Family or cultural resistance to your changes

**Support system development** ensures you have people and resources to help you maintain motivation and accountability for your life vision while providing reality testing when needed.

Support categories to develop:

- Emotional support: People who encourage your growth and provide comfort during difficulties

- Practical support: People who can help with concrete needs and problem-solving

- Accountability support: People who help you stay committed to your goals and values

- Professional support: Therapists, coaches, or consultants who provide specialized guidance

- Community support: Groups or organizations aligned with your values and goals

**Progress Monitoring and Adjustment**

**Regular life assessment** helps you track progress toward your vision while remaining flexible about adjusting goals as you continue growing and learning about yourself.

Monthly check-in questions:

- Am I living according to my values or reverting to old survival patterns?

- What progress have I made toward my goals this month?

- What obstacles or challenges have I encountered?

- How has my vision of the future shifted based on new experiences?

- What support or resources do I need for continued progress?

**Celebration and appreciation practice** helps you recognize and enjoy the positive changes you're creating rather than focusing exclusively on remaining problems or future goals.

Weekly appreciation exercise:

- What evidence of healing and growth did I notice this week?

- What choices did I make based on authentic values rather than trauma fears?

- What relationships, activities, or experiences brought me genuine satisfaction?

- How did I handle challenges differently than I would have before healing?

- What am I grateful for about my current life and future possibilities?

**The Horizon of Possibility**

Building a life beyond trauma represents more than recovery from past wounds—it's about discovering and creating possibilities that trauma may have hidden but never destroyed. The person you become through healing is not who you would have been without trauma, but rather someone who carries both the strength that survival required and the openness that healing makes possible.

This integration of survival strength with authentic living creates unique capacities for depth, empathy, resilience, and meaning-making that can become gifts not just to yourself but to everyone whose life you touch. Your healing journey becomes part of your contribution to the world's healing, demonstrating that growth and transformation remain possible even after the most difficult circumstances.

The life you build beyond trauma won't be perfect or free from all difficulties. But it can be authentic in ways that weren't possible during survival mode, meaningful in ways that feel genuine to your core values, and satisfying in ways that don't depend on avoiding all potential problems or managing other people's responses to your authentic self.

Most importantly, the skills, insights, and internal changes that schema therapy creates become resources you can use throughout your life as new challenges and opportunities arise. The same intelligence that helped you survive trauma and commit to healing can guide you in creating whatever life feels true and meaningful to you.

Your story of healing becomes part of the larger human story of resilience, growth, and the remarkable capacity to transform pain into wisdom, isolation into connection, and survival into authentic living. This transformation doesn't erase what happened to you, but it proves that what happened to you doesn't have to determine what happens next.

**Building Your Future Foundations**

- Post-traumatic growth creates possibilities for positive changes that might not have occurred without the healing journey

- Maintaining progress requires ongoing schema awareness and skill practice rather than just completing therapy

- Sustained recovery involves continued growth and development long after formal treatment ends

- Life planning should incorporate authentic values and goals rather than trauma-driven limitations

- Support systems and professional resources provide ongoing foundations for continued development

- Regular assessment and adjustment help maintain progress while allowing for natural life changes

- The ultimate goal is authentic living that honors both your survival strength and your growth potential

# References

(1) National Center for Mental Health Promotion and Youth Violence Prevention. (2012). Childhood trauma and its effects on healthy development. *Substance Abuse and Mental Health Services Administration*.

(2) Felitti, V. J., Anda, R. F., Nordenberg, D., Williamson, D. F., Spitz, A. M., Edwards, V., ... & Marks, J. S. (1998). Relationship of childhood abuse and household dysfunction to many of the leading causes of death in adults: The Adverse Childhood Experiences (ACE) Study. *American Journal of Preventive Medicine*, 14(4), 245-258.

(3) van der Kolk, B. A., McFarlane, A. C., & Weisaeth, L. (Eds.). (2007). *Traumatic stress: The effects of overwhelming experience on mind, body, and society*. The Guilford Press.

(4) Teicher, M. H., Andersen, S. L., Polcari, A., Anderson, C. M., & Navalta, C. P. (2002). Developmental neurobiology of childhood stress and trauma. *Psychiatric Clinics of North America*, 25(2), 397-426.

(5) van der Kolk, B. A., McFarlane, A. C., & Weisaeth, L. (Eds.). (2007). *Traumatic stress: The effects of overwhelming experience on mind, body, and society*. The Guilford Press.

(6) Herman, J. L. (1992). *Complex PTSD: A syndrome in survivors of prolonged and repeated trauma. Journal of Traumatic Stress*, 5(3), 377-391.

(7) Young, J. E., Klosko, J. S., & Weishaar, M. E. (2003). *Schema therapy: A practitioner's guide*. The Guilford Press.

(8) Teicher, M. H., Andersen, S. L., Polcari, A., Anderson, C. M., & Navalta, C. P. (2002). Developmental neurobiology of

childhood stress and trauma. *Psychiatric Clinics of North America*, 25(2), 397-426.

(9) Schmidt, N. B., Joiner, T. E., Young, J. E., & Telch, M. J. (1995). The Schema Questionnaire: Investigation of psychometric properties and the hierarchical structure of a measure of maladaptive schemata. *Cognitive Therapy and Research*, 19(3), 295-321.

(10) Arntz, A., & van Genderen, H. (2009). *Schema therapy for borderline personality disorder*. John Wiley & Sons.

(11) Giesen-Bloo, J., van Dyck, R., Spinhoven, P., van Tilburg, W., Dirksen, C., van Asselt, T., ... & Arntz, A. (2006). Outpatient psychotherapy for borderline personality disorder: Randomized trial of schema-focused therapy vs transference-focused psychotherapy. *Archives of General Psychiatry*, 63(6), 649-658.

(12) Linehan, M. M. (1993). *Skills training manual for treating borderline personality disorder*. The Guilford Press.

(13) Neff, K. D. (2003). Self-compassion: An alternative conceptualization of a healthy attitude toward oneself. *Self and Identity*, 2(2), 85-101.

(14) Kabat-Zinn, J. (1994). *Wherever you go, there you are: Mindfulness meditation in everyday life*. Hyperion.

(15) Siegel, D. J. (2012). *The developing mind: How relationships and the brain interact to shape who we are* (2nd ed.). The Guilford Press.

(16) Young, J. E. (1990). *Cognitive therapy for personality disorders: A schema-focused approach*. Professional Resource Exchange.

(17) Beck, A. T., Freeman, A., & Davis, D. D. (2004). *Cognitive therapy of personality disorders* (2nd ed.). The Guilford Press.

(18) Kellogg, S. H., & Young, J. E. (2006). Schema therapy for borderline personality disorder. *Journal of Clinical Psychology*, 62(4), 445-458.

(19) Rafaeli, E., Bernstein, D. P., & Young, J. E. (2011). *Schema therapy: Distinctive features*. Routledge.

(20) van Vreeswijk, M., Broersen, J., & Nadort, M. (Eds.). (2012). *The Wiley-Blackwell handbook of schema therapy: Theory, research, and practice*. John Wiley & Sons.

(21) Farrell, J. M., Shaw, I. A., & Webber, M. A. (2009). A schema-focused approach to group psychotherapy for outpatients with borderline personality disorder: A randomized controlled trial. *Journal of Behavior Therapy and Experimental Psychiatry*, 40(2), 317-328.

(22) Bamelis, L. L., Evers, S. M., Spinhoven, P., & Arntz, A. (2014). Results of a multicenter randomized controlled trial of the clinical effectiveness of schema therapy for personality disorders. *American Journal of Psychiatry*, 171(3), 305-322.

(23) Jacob, G. A., & Arntz, A. (2013). Schema therapy for personality disorders—A review. *International Journal of Cognitive Therapy*, 6(3), 171-185.

(24) Sempértegui, G. A., Karreman, A., Arntz, A., & Bekker, M. H. (2013). Schema therapy for borderline personality disorder: A comprehensive review of its empirical foundations, effectiveness and implementation possibilities. *Clinical Psychology Review*, 33(3), 426-447.

(25) Neff, K. D. (2011). *Self-compassion: The proven power of being kind to yourself*. William Morrow Paperbacks.

(26) Gilbert, P. (2009). *The compassionate mind: A new approach to life's challenges*. New Harbinger Publications.

(27) Porges, S. W. (2011). *The polyvagal theory: Neurophysiological foundations of emotions, attachment, communication, and self-regulation*. W. W. Norton & Company.

(28) Cozolino, L. (2014). *The neuroscience of human relationships: Attachment and the developing social brain* (2nd ed.). W. W. Norton & Company.

(29) Briere, J., & Scott, C. (2015). *Principles of trauma therapy: A guide to symptoms, evaluation, and treatment* (2nd ed.). SAGE Publications.

(30) Courtois, C. A., & Ford, J. D. (2009). *Treating complex traumatic stress disorders: An evidence-based guide*. The Guilford Press.

(31) Young, J. E., Klosko, J. S., & Weishaar, M. E. (2003). *Schema therapy: A practitioner's guide*. The Guilford Press.

(32) Arntz, A., & van Genderen, H. (2009). *Schema therapy for borderline personality disorder*. John Wiley & Sons.

(33) Edwards, D. J., & Arntz, A. (2012). Schema therapy in historical perspective. In M. van Vreeswijk, J. Broersen, & M. Nadort (Eds.), *The Wiley-Blackwell handbook of schema therapy: Theory, research, and practice* (pp. 3-26). John Wiley & Sons.

(34) Smucker, M. R., & Dancu, C. V. (1999). *Cognitive-behavioral treatment for adult survivors of childhood trauma: Imagery rescripting and reprocessing.* Jason Aronson.

(35) Hackmann, A., Bennett-Levy, J., & Holmes, E. A. (2011). *Oxford guide to imagery in cognitive therapy.* Oxford University Press.

(36) Malkinson, R., Rubin, S. S., & Witztum, E. (2006). *Therapeutic intervention and human response to loss: Coping with dying, death, and bereavement.* Death Studies, 30(8), 715-738.

(37) Safran, J. D., & Muran, J. C. (2000). *Negotiating the therapeutic alliance: A relational treatment guide.* The Guilford Press.

(38) Gelso, C. J., & Hayes, J. A. (2007). *Countertransference and the therapist's inner experience: Perils and possibilities.* Lawrence Erlbaum Associates.

(39) Courtois, C. A. (2004). Complex trauma, complex reactions: Assessment and treatment. *Psychotherapy: Theory, Research, Practice, Training,* 41(4), 412-425.

(40) Cozolino, L. (2014). *The neuroscience of human relationships: Attachment and the developing social brain* (2nd ed.). W. W. Norton & Company.

(41) Linehan, M. M. (1993). *Cognitive-behavioral treatment of borderline personality disorder.* The Guilford Press.

(42) Beck, J. S. (2011). *Cognitive behavior therapy: Basics and beyond* (2nd ed.). The Guilford Press.

(43) Hayes, S. C., Strosahl, K. D., & Wilson, K. G. (2012). *Acceptance and commitment therapy: The process and practice of mindful change* (2nd ed.). The Guilford Press.

(44) Wolpe, J. (1958). *Psychotherapy by reciprocal inhibition.* Stanford University Press.

(45) Bandura, A. (1977). *Social learning theory.* Prentice Hall.

(46) Shapiro, F. (2001). *Eye movement desensitization and reprocessing (EMDR): Basic principles, protocols, and procedures* (2nd ed.). The Guilford Press.

(47) Levine, P. A. (2010). *In an unspoken voice: How the body releases trauma and restores goodness.* North Atlantic Books.

(48) van der Kolk, B. A. (2014). *The body keeps the score: Brain, mind, and body in the healing of trauma.* Viking.

(49) Porges, S. W. (2011). *The polyvagal theory: Neurophysiological foundations of emotions, attachment, communication, and self-regulation.* W. W. Norton & Company.

(50) Rothschild, B. (2000). *The body remembers: The psychophysiology of trauma and trauma treatment.* W. W. Norton & Company.

(51) Ogden, P., Minton, K., & Pain, C. (2006). *Trauma and the body: A sensorimotor approach to psychotherapy.* W. W. Norton & Company.

(52) Farrell, J. M., Shaw, I. A., & Webber, M. A. (2009). A schema-focused approach to group psychotherapy for outpatients with borderline personality disorder: A

randomized controlled trial. *Journal of Behavior Therapy and Experimental Psychiatry*, 40(2), 317-328.

(53) Yalom, I. D., & Leszcz, M. (2005). *The theory and practice of group psychotherapy* (5th ed.). Basic Books.

(54) Rutan, J. S., Stone, W. N., & Shay, J. J. (2007). *Psychodynamic group psychotherapy* (4th ed.). The Guilford Press.

(55) McGoldrick, M., Giordano, J., & Garcia-Preto, N. (Eds.). (2005). *Ethnicity and family therapy* (3rd ed.). The Guilford Press.

(56) Sue, D. W., & Sue, D. (2015). *Counseling the culturally diverse: Theory and practice* (7th ed.). John Wiley & Sons.

(57) Carter, R. T. (2007). Racism and psychological and emotional injury: Recognizing and assessing race-based traumatic stress. *The Counseling Psychologist*, 35(1), 13-105.

(58) Brave Heart, M. Y. H. (2003). The historical trauma response among natives and its relationship with substance abuse: A Lakota illustration. *Journal of Psychoactive Drugs*, 35(1), 7-13.

(59) Comas-Díaz, L., & Jacobsen, F. M. (1991). Ethnocultural transference and countertransference in the therapeutic dyad. *American Journal of Orthopsychiatry*, 61(3), 392-402.

(60) Hays, P. A. (2008). *Addressing cultural complexities in practice: Assessment, diagnosis, and therapy* (2nd ed.). American Psychological Association.

(61) Tedeschi, R. G., & Calhoun, L. G. (2004). Posttraumatic growth: Conceptual foundations and empirical evidence. *Psychological Inquiry*, 15(1), 1-18.

(62) Joseph, S. (2011). *What doesn't kill us: The new psychology of posttraumatic growth*. Basic Books.

(63) Calhoun, L. G., & Tedeschi, R. G. (2013). *Posttraumatic growth in clinical practice*. Routledge.

(64) Janoff-Bulman, R. (2004). Posttraumatic growth: Three explanatory models. *Psychological Inquiry*, 15(1), 30-34.

(65) Park, C. L. (2010). Making sense of the meaning literature: An integrative review of meaning making and its effects on adjustment to stressful life events. *Psychological Bulletin*, 136(2), 257-301.

(66) Bonanno, G. A. (2004). Loss, trauma, and human resilience: Have we underestimated the human capacity to thrive after extremely aversive events? *American Psychologist*, 59(1), 20-28.

(67) Masten, A. S. (2001). Ordinary magic: Resilience processes in development. *American Psychologist*, 56(3), 227-238.

(68) Rutter, M. (2012). Resilience as a dynamic concept. *Development and Psychopathology*, 24(2), 335-344.

(69) Southwick, S. M., & Charney, D. S. (2012). *Resilience: The science of mastering life's greatest challenges*. Cambridge University Press.

(70) Duckworth, A. L. (2016). *Grit: The power of passion and perseverance*. Scribner.

(71) Brown, B. (2010). *The gifts of imperfection: Let go of who you think you're supposed to be and embrace who you are*. Hazelden Publishing.

(72) Kabat-Zinn, J. (2013). *Full catastrophe living: Using the wisdom of your body and mind to face stress, pain, and illness* (2nd ed.). Bantam Books.

(73) Seligman, M. E. P. (2011). *Flourish: A visionary new understanding of happiness and well-being*. Free Press.

(74) Frankl, V. E. (2006). *Man's search for meaning*. Beacon Press. (Original work published 1946)

(75) Hayes, S. C., Strosahl, K. D., & Wilson, K. G. (2012). *Acceptance and commitment therapy: The process and practice of mindful change* (2nd ed.). The Guilford Press.

www.ingramcontent.com/pod-product-compliance
Lightning Source LLC
Chambersburg PA
CBHW050501270326
41927CB00009B/1842